A Philosophical Framework for Psychotherapy Integration

In this thought-provoking work, Yael Peri Herzovich and Aner Govrin challenge the long-standing rivalry between psychoanalysis and other psychotherapeutic approaches, particularly cognitive-behavioral therapy. They address a fundamental question: How can we facilitate genuine dialogue between these dominant psychotherapy schools?

Drawing on philosophical concepts such as Derrida's notion of hospitality, Hegel's dialectics, and Gadamer's dialogical approach, the authors provide a new philosophical framework for encountering the "other" in psychotherapy integration. This book examines the barriers to integration and explores how hospitality, dialectics, and dialogue processes can facilitate openness between schools while preserving their unique identities. Through engaging historical analysis and practical demonstrations, the authors show how opposing approaches can enrich each other, leading to more effective treatment possibilities.

Offering a fresh perspective on the potential for integration and mutual influence between these two major psychotherapy schools, while honouring the unique contributions of each school, this book is essential reading for psychotherapists, psychoanalysts, psychologists, and students of mental health.

Yael Peri Herzovich, PhD, is a clinical psychologist who practices, teaches, and researches from an integrative stance in psychotherapy. She lectures and supervises in the "Ogen (Anchor) - a Program for Training in Integration Based Psychotherapy" at "Mifrasim (Sails) - Institute for Psychotherapy Research and Training" in the School of Behavioral Sciences at the Academic College of Tel-Aviv Yaffo, and serves as Executive Editor of Routledge Introductions to Contemporary Psychoanalysis.

Aner Govrin, PhD, is a clinical psychologist, psychoanalyst, and philosopher. He is head of the doctoral track "Psychoanalysis and Hermeneutics" at Bar-Ilan University, a member of Tel-Aviv Institute for Contemporary Psychoanalysis, and editor of the Routledge Introductions to Contemporary Psychoanalysis series. His last book *How Philosophy Changed Psychoanalysis from Naive Realism to Postmodernism* was published by Routledge in 2025.

Philosophy and Psychoanalysis Book Series
Series Editor
Jon Mills

Philosophy and Psychoanalysis is dedicated to current developments and cutting-edge research in the philosophical sciences, phenomenology, hermeneutics, existentialism, logic, semiotics, cultural studies, social criticism, and the humanities that engage and enrich psychoanalytic thought through philosophical rigor. With the philosophical turn in psychoanalysis comes a new era of theoretical research that revisits past paradigms while invigorating new approaches to theoretical, historical, contemporary, and applied psychoanalysis. No subject or discipline is immune from psychoanalytic reflection within a philosophical context including psychology, sociology, anthropology, politics, the arts, religion, science, culture, physics, and the nature of morality. Philosophical approaches to psychoanalysis may stimulate new areas of knowledge that have conceptual and applied value beyond the consulting room reflective of greater society at large. In the spirit of pluralism, *Philosophy and Psychoanalysis* is open to any theoretical school in philosophy and psychoanalysis that offers novel, scholarly, and important insights in the way we come to understand our world.
Titles in this series:

Monstrosity and the Psychoanalytic Dimensions of the Uncanny
Rodrigo Gonsalves

Selected Essays of Ladson Hinton
Psychoanalytic and Existential Reflections on Shame and Temporality
Hessel Willemsen

A Psycho-Political Analysis of Netanyahu's Israel
The Israeli Anxiety
Itzhak Benyamini

A Philosophical Framework for Psychotherapy Integration
Psychoanalysis Meets Otherness
Yael Peri Herzovich and Aner Govrin

A Philosophical Framework for Psychotherapy Integration

Psychoanalysis Meets Otherness

Yael Peri Herzovich and Aner Govrin

Routledge
Taylor & Francis Group

LONDON AND NEW YORK

Designed cover image: Getty Images

First published 2026
by Routledge
4 Park Square, Milton Park, Abingdon, Oxon OX14 4RN

and by Routledge
605 Third Avenue, New York, NY 10158

Routledge is an imprint of the Taylor & Francis Group, an informa business

© 2026 Yael Peri Herzovich and Aner Govrin

For Product Safety Concerns and Information please contact our EU
representative GPSR@taylorandfrancis.com. Taylor & Francis Verlag GmbH,
Kaufingerstraße 24, 80331 München, Germany.

British Library Cataloguing-in-Publication Data
A catalogue record for this book is available from the British Library

ISBN: 978-1-041-00088-4 (hbk)
ISBN: 978-1-041-00086-0 (pbk)
ISBN: 978-1-003-60810-3 (ebk)

DOI: 10.4324/9781003608103

Typeset in Times New Roman
by codeMantra

Contents

Acknowledgments

We are profoundly grateful to Jon Mills, the series editor of *Philosophy and Psychoanalysis*, for his support and for including our work in this distinguished collection. We also extend our sincere appreciation to Routledge for embracing this project within their esteemed series, which provides an interdisciplinary platform for exploring the rich connections between these fields.

Parts of this book were written as part of a doctoral study undertaken by Yael Peri Herzovich at Bar-Ilan University in the Program for Hermeneutics and Cultural Studies, with Aner Govrin serving as supervisor. We are deeply grateful to the Israel Science Foundation for their generous support: the research grant (1392/19) that made this investigation possible, as well as the workshop grant that enabled us to organize the international research workshop "A Psychodynamic therapist and a CBT therapist meet on a plane… – Psychotherapy Integration as Hospitality" at Bar-Ilan University, Ramat-Gan, Israel, on September 20–22, 2022. This workshop was fundamental in inspiring the conception of this book.

We wish to express our gratitude to the steering committee of the workshop: Prof. Sharon Ziv-Beiman, Prof. Golan Shahar, and Prof. Eva Gilboa-Schechtman, whose guidance was instrumental in shaping the workshop's direction and success. We are equally indebted to all the esteemed workshop participants whose valuable contributions and dialogues significantly influenced the ideas presented in this work: Prof. Jon Mills, Dr. Monica Luci, Prof. Stephen Frosh, Prof. Jonathan Huppert, Prof. Golan Shahar, Prof. Eva Gilboa-Schechtman, Prof. Eshkol Rafaeli, Prof. Idan M Aderka, Nili Cohen Aaronson, and Dr. Hilit Brodsky.

We extend our appreciation to the *British Journal of Psychotherapy* (BJP), John Wiley & Sons for publishing two articles that contributed to this book: "Psychoanalysis and CBT: From Rivalry to Hospitality in Psychotherapy Integration" and "Dialectical Integration: The Case of Psychoanalysis and Cognitive Behavioral Therapy." We also thank Frontiers for publishing "Psychoanalysis and Interdisciplinarity with Non-analytic Psychotherapeutic Approaches Through the Prism of Dialectics." We are grateful to both journals for granting permission to incorporate this material into the present work.

Yael Peri Herzovich and Aner Govrin

*Introduction

When Therapists Cross Theoretical Borders

Aner Govrin and Yael Peri Herzovich

On a warm September morning in 2022, an unusual three-days gathering took place at Bar-Ilan University in Ramat-Gan, Israel. Twelve distinguished psychotherapists and scholars from different parts of the world came together for what might be described as an experimental encounter. The workshop, playfully titled "A Psychodynamic therapist and a CBT therapist meet on a plane... – Psychotherapy Integration as Hospitality," was not just another academic conference. It was, in many ways, an unprecedented experiment in therapeutic dialogue.

What made this gathering unique was its deliberate bringing together of clinicians who rarely find themselves in the same room: deeply committed psychodynamic practitioners, committed cognitive-behavioral therapists, and integrative psychotherapists. These groups, despite sharing the common goal of helping people through psychological means, often operate in parallel universes, rarely engaging in meaningful dialogue with one another. When they do meet, their encounters are usually marked by skepticism, criticism, or even hostility.

The workshop, sponsored by the Israel Science Foundation (ISF), was inspired by Jacques Derrida's concept of hospitality – a philosophical framework that suggests a way of engaging with otherness while maintaining one's own identity. Just as hospitality involves opening one's home to strangers while retaining control over the threshold, we envisioned a space where different therapeutic approaches could meet, interact, and learn from each other without losing their essential character.

The participants represented a remarkable cross-section of therapeutic approaches. From the psychodynamic tradition came **Stephen Frosh** (Birkbeck, University of London) and **Jon Mills** (University of Essex). **Idan M. Aderka** (University of Haifa) and **Jonathan Huppert** (The Hebrew University of Jerusalem) brought their expertise in cognitive-behavioral approaches. The integration perspective was powerfully represented by **Eshkol Rafaeli** (Bar-Ilan University), who has done groundbreaking work in schema therapy. **Eva Gilboa-Schechtman** (Bar-Ilan University) contributed her insights on active exploration and belief modification, while **Nilly Aronson** (The Center for the Treatment and Research of Autism) shared her patient-focused approach. **Monica Luci**, a private practitioner from Rome, offered a unique perspective bridging psychoanalysis and analytical psychology, while **Hilit Brodsky** (Bar-Ilan University) explored the relationship between home and the unknown in therapeutic practice.

DOI: 10.4324/9781003608103-1

Golan Shahar (Ben-Gurion University of the Negev) brought his expertise in existential approaches and their integration with psychological science. The workshop was organized by the authors of this book: **Yael Peri Herzovich** (Bar-Ilan University), an integrative therapist who combines psychodynamic and cognitive-behavioral approaches in both practice and research, and **Aner Govrin** (Bar-Ilan University), a psychoanalyst and philosopher who has published extensively on the philosophy of psychoanalysis and its intersection with other fields of knowledge.

The workshop was structured around three main themes that unfolded over the three days:

First, we explored the fundamental encounter with the psychotherapeutic "other" – examining existing meetings between different approaches, identifying barriers to mutual influence, and discussing the necessity of dialogue. Stephen Frosh's presentation "Feeling at Home with Psychoanalysis" and Eva Gilboa-Schechtman's "Homebase: Active Exploration and Modifying Beliefs About the Self" exemplified the rich diversity of perspectives brought to this theme.

Second, we investigated the multiple faces of mutual influence across theory, practice, and research. Eshkol Rafaeli's exploration of schema therapy as a model of integration and Monica Luci's examination of psychoanalytic approaches to human rights violations demonstrated how different theoretical frameworks can inform and enrich each other.

Third, we grappled with the tension between monolithic approaches and integration – perhaps the most challenging theme of all. Key questions emerged: How important are monolithic approaches in contemporary psychotherapy? What value might they gain from influence by other approaches? How can we maintain the creative tension between theoretical purity and pluralistic integration?

These themes led to several crucial areas of inquiry that dominated our discussions:

1 The necessity of mutual influence between different schools of psychotherapy, particularly for monolithic approaches. We questioned whether maintaining pure theoretical approaches remains valuable in contemporary psychotherapy and how such approaches might benefit from cross-pollination while maintaining their essential character.

2 The identification and analysis of barriers that impede mutual influence between different approaches. Participants explored what obstacles continue to exist in creating dialogue between adherents of different therapeutic schools and what elements might be missing in current integration efforts.

3 The complex relationship between theory, technique, and research, and how these elements affect the potential for mutual influence. We examined whether theoretical loyalty can coexist with practical flexibility and how research might bridge gaps between different approaches.

4 The practical applications of mutual influence through the lens of hospitality. Could openness to "foreign" ideas generate novel therapeutic insights? What approaches might help reduce resistance and promote dialogue between different schools of thought?

The metaphor of home and hospitality ran deep throughout the workshop. Golan Shahar challenged the very notion with his presentation "Home is where the patient is (Or: Why the term 'therapeutic home' is not valid)," while Hilit Brodsky explored the idea that "Home is where the unknown is." These seemingly contradictory perspectives created a rich tapestry of dialogue about what it means to have a theoretical home while remaining open to other approaches.

The final roundtable discussions attempted to capture these emerging insights and prepare a summary document that would serve as a foundation for future dialogue. The discussions revealed both the challenges and the potential of therapeutic integration, suggesting that perhaps the way forward lies not in dissolving theoretical differences but in learning how to engage with them productively.

This workshop, which forms the foundation for the book you are about to read, demonstrated that meaningful dialogue across theoretical boundaries is possible when approached with the right framework and attitude. The concepts of hospitality and integration that emerged from these discussions offer a new way of thinking about how different therapeutic approaches might interact while maintaining their unique identities.

As you proceed through the chapters of this book, you will encounter many of the ideas that were first explored during those three days in Ramat-Gan. Some will feel familiar, others strange, and still others might challenge your fundamental assumptions about psychotherapy. We invite you to approach these ideas with the same spirit of hospitality that characterized our workshop – as a guest willing to explore new theoretical territories while remaining grounded in your own therapeutic home.

This book emerges from that remarkable gathering in Ramat-Gan, but it reaches far beyond those three days of dialogue. While the workshop served as a living laboratory for the concept of therapeutic hospitality, this volume expands and deepens those initial explorations, offering a philosophical framework for understanding and facilitating integration between different therapeutic approaches, particularly psychoanalysis and cognitive-behavioral therapy (CBT).

At its heart, this book addresses a fundamental question: What might facilitate a genuine encounter between proponents of these dominant psychotherapeutic methodologies? While the field of psychotherapy integration has long focused on developing coherent models that incorporate multiple approaches, relatively little attention has been paid to understanding and addressing the deep-seated resistances to integration among adherents of monolithic approaches. Our book fills this crucial gap by providing a philosophical, epistemological, and ontological foundation for encountering the "other" in psychotherapy integration.

The journey unfolds across five chapters, each building upon the others while exploring distinct aspects of this challenge.

In Chapter 1, "Resistance to Integration: Psychoanalysis and the Fear of Otherness" we confront a puzzling phenomenon: despite historical precedent – including Freud's own use of what we might today call behavioral activation – mainstream psychoanalysis has failed to produce a community of practitioners open to integration with CBT. The chapter offers a fascinating exploration of five key barriers to integration, from identity threats to the power of ignorance, while suggesting practical ways forward.

Chapter 2, "Psychoanalysis and CBT: From Rivalry to Hospitality in Psychotherapy Integration," introduces our central theoretical framework. Drawing on Derrida's concept of hospitality, we explore how therapeutic approaches might maintain their distinct identities while genuinely engaging with other perspectives. Just as hospitality involves both welcoming the stranger and maintaining the integrity of one's home, we argue that therapeutic integration requires both openness to other approaches and preservation of one's theoretical foundations.

In Chapter 3, "Dialectical Integration: The Case of Psychoanalysis and Cognitive-Behavioral Therapy," we take an unexpected turn by applying Hegelian dialectics to understand how different psychotherapies, despite their apparent antagonism, profoundly influence each other through unconscious processes. Through detailed analysis of developments like Hartmann's ego psychology and Young's schema therapy, we reveal how theoretical advances often involve the reintegration of previously rejected ideas from other approaches.

Chapter 4, "Psychoanalysis and Interdisciplinarity with Nonanalytic Psychotherapeutic Approaches Through the Prism of Dialectics," challenges the common view of psychoanalysis as an isolationist discipline. Through examination of three pivotal developments – empathy in self-psychology, short-term dynamic psychotherapy, and mentalization-based therapy – we demonstrate how psychoanalysis has evolved through dialectical engagement with other approaches while maintaining its essential character.

Chapter 5, "Fusion of Horizons in Psychotherapy Integration: A Dialogue Between Psychoanalysis and Cognitive-Behavioral Therapy," draws on Gadamer's hermeneutics to propose that the very differences that seem to block dialogue between therapeutic approaches might actually hold the key to integration. We explore how the "fusion of horizons" between different therapeutic traditions can lead to deeper understanding while preserving each approach's unique identity.

What makes this book unique is not just its theoretical sophistication but its practical implications. Throughout these chapters, we demonstrate how philosophical concepts like hospitality, dialectics, and dialogue can help practitioners engage with other approaches while maintaining their therapeutic identities. We offer not just theoretical frameworks but practical strategies for fostering integration while respecting theoretical differences.

This book is written for a diverse audience – from students and therapists-in-training to experienced practitioners and researchers. Whether you identify primarily with psychoanalysis, CBT, or an integrative approach, you'll find here new ways of thinking about therapeutic integration and your own relationship to different therapeutic traditions.

Ultimately, we hope this work contributes to shifting the very terms of debate about psychotherapy integration. Rather than asking whether integration is possible or desirable, we invite readers to consider what conditions make genuine encounter between different therapeutic traditions both challenging and potentially transformative.

Chapter 1

Resistance to Integration
Psychoanalysis and the Fear of Otherness

Aner Govrin

Mainstream psychoanalysis has not fostered a community of analysts committed to integrating it with cognitive-behavioral therapy (CBT). This failure is a surprising lacuna given that several mainstream psychoanalysts, including Freud, have always sought to combine cognitive therapeutic principles and psychoanalysis. Their ideas, however, did not resonate in the community. Here I introduce these efforts, including a case in which Freud used what would today be characterized as behavioral activation (BA) technique in treating a patient with obsession thoughts. The chapter offers five reasons for the failure of such integration: identity (a threat to psychoanalysis's uniqueness), the psychoanalytic narrative (nonanalytic elements are strident within psychoanalysis coherent narratives), accept or reject all (the impossibility of accepting a part without accepting the whole), a theory under siege (criticism against the discipline causes suspiciousness and a defensive approach), and ignorance (psychodynamic psychotherapists simply don't know enough about CBT). The chapter locates these reasons in the shared social need to preserve identity, distinctiveness, and singularity. It argues for the importance of integration and discusses how it may be encouraged despite resistance.

Introduction

Like religion, science is susceptible to the biases embedded in all social activity: fanaticism and in-group preference. It has always developed through social networks. Like any other club, it has its dogmatism and fundamentalism, functionaries and visionaries, loyalties to charismatic leaders, and harsh insider and outsider politics (Laudan et al., 1986).

Mainstream psychoanalysis continues to erect substantial barriers to external influences. This is strongly manifested by its general reluctance to be influenced by active therapeutic techniques, such as CBT. This refusal is in sharp contrast to a robust and frequently noticed rationale for why psychoanalysts should indeed have sought CBT's integration within their overarching theory.

In the first part of this chapter, we shall see that many analysts within the establishment (including Freud) combined psychodynamic and what we would now call

DOI: 10.4324/9781003608103-2

cognitive-behavioral techniques. Integrating psychoanalysis and CBT was often used in special cases in which the sole reliance on psychoanalysis was not effective enough for various reasons. The second part of this chapter indicates five reasons to explain the fact that such integration has never occurred: identity (a threat to psychoanalysis' uniqueness), the psychoanalytic narrative (nonanalytic elements are strident within psychoanalysis coherent narratives), accept or reject all (the impossibility of incorporating a part without accepting the whole), a theory under siege (criticism against the discipline causes suspiciousness and a defensive approach), and ignorance (psychodynamic psychotherapists know little about CBT). The third part suggests that alongside one-school community should exist a small community of analysts dedicated to integration.

Govrin (2016) posit that sectarianism, indoctrination, and resistance to change for which psychoanalysis is sometimes berated are very characteristic of other scientific communities. There is a remarkable similarity between the ways psychoanalytic and scientific communities claim knowledge. Indeed, the questions raised regarding the psychoanalytic community's refusal to incorporate aspects of CBT and other active techniques are the very same questions raised by philosophers of science when they investigate indoctrination and the rejection of scientific truth in different scientific communities (Harman & Dietrich, 2013; Levenson, 2015; Musser, 2016; Wootton, 2016).

For post-positivist philosophers of science, such as Kuhn, Laudan, Lakatos, and Thagard (for a comprehensive summary of such approaches, see Laudan et al., 1986), scientific paradigms and research traditions, once adopted, are rarely, if ever, rejected solely because new empirical findings raise doubts as to their validity (Lakatos, 1978). According to post-positivist philosophers of science, contradictory findings change scientific theories far less than is commonly believed. Aesthetic considerations, doctrinal beliefs, and other, not necessarily empirically based considerations play an essential role in the judgment of scientific theories and research traditions.

Like other communities, psychotherapeutic communities tend to isolate themselves from each other. There is a Gestalt community, psychodynamic community, family therapy community, humanistic therapy community, mindfulness community, and many others. These communities seem to manage in mutual isolation, each developing its own ideas. The integration movement is another community that attempts to bring these different approaches together in many ways. Its activity is mainly outside these one-school orientations, and it has a journal, annual conference, and organization (SEPI).

Of course, the clear-cut boundaries between "us" and "them" are always contested, employing elaborate explanations concerning the incompatibility at hand – for example, the response of conservatives in the CBT community to mindfulness-based cognitive therapy (MBCT). CBT loyalists found that incorporating Zen Buddhism, which they regarded as being based on mystical assumptions, by a rationally and scientifically based psychotherapy was to stretch CBT to foreign worldviews. For conservatives, it was hard to accept that the teachings of Thich Nhat Hanh, for instance, should be incorporated into an approach that was proud of its rationality and close adherence to the scientific method (Harrington & Pickles, 2009; Hofmann & Asmundson, 2008; Leahy, 2008). In their criticism, they went so far as to compare practitioners of MBCT (Mindfulness-Based Cognitive Therapy) to Vulcans, who feature in the sci-fi TV series Star Trek and use mind control (i.e., meditation and strict adherence to logic) (David, 2014). Those in favor of the approach – often titled "Third Wave CBT" (Hayes & Hofmann, 2017) – responded to the criticism by completely repudiating the mystical foundations of mindfulness and stressing the similarity between it and traditional CBT techniques. The host theory can be said, disowned the new idea, and created its own type of integration through what I once referred to as integration by conversion (Govrin, 2016).

The desire to maintain the purity of psychoanalysis and the refusal to allow external influences have a long history. A famous historical example is the hostile reaction of Anna Freud and her supporters to the theories of Melanie Klein. Other examples are the renowned opposition of the psychoanalytic establishment to the ideas of Karen Horney and Heinz Kohut. Also, the conservative opposition (Blass & Carmeli, 2007) to neuropsychoanalysis and infant observation research (Green, 2000), arguing that their findings are too remote from psychoanalysis's original objective uncovering of the patient's unconscious.

But the attitude of mainstream psychoanalysis to other therapeutic methods was even harsher. It seldom referred to them, and when it did, it reflected a dismissive tone.

Kohut, for example, was critical of nonanalytic and non-interpretive psychotherapeutic counseling. He compares such methods to a repairman who knows nothing about watches but manages to get his old alarm clock to work again simply by cleaning and oiling the internal mechanism:

> There is no need to spell out the analogy between the so-called watchmaker and the practitioners of certain kinds of psychotherapy – except, I think, that my so called watchmaker had a higher percentage of successes and knew more about what he was doing than most of the psychotherapists who borrow one or the other insight or technical rule from psychoanalysis and apply it without understanding.
> (Kohut, 1978, p. 525)

Kohut's contempt for non-psychoanalytic approaches determined psychoanalysis superiority over other methods of treatment.

In all probability, conservatism both helped maintain its identity and, at the same time, kept psychoanalysis isolated and detached, giving it a reputation of being sectarian and exclusive (Bornstein, 2001).

The purists were always an important voice in the psychoanalytic community. Nevertheless, those purists suffered many defeats. In fact, psychoanalysis did not maintain its original form throughout the years, and today it does not resemble the classical version that Freud and his close followers have developed. Even if it successfully warded off variously theoretical contestations and innovations, it was nevertheless not immune to the changing times massive social and cultural transformations. Despite tremendous opposition, two communities that "married out" – neuropsychoanalysis and infant observation research – continue to be active and vibrant, opting to incorporate findings from their unique methodologies into psychoanalytic theory and practice (Rustin, 2013; Seligman, 2018; Stern, 2010). Neuropsychoanalysis has also established an international organization with worldwide local branches and a journal of its own (Yovell et al., 2015).

Using Elements of CBT within Psychoanalysis

Techniques from non-analytic theories had already appeared quite prominently in its earliest days. Let us start with Freud. There are many components in his theory and practice which incorporate the elements of CBT. To illustrate this, I discuss in detail the case of Bruno Walter, where Freud can use, in effect, Behavioral Activation (BA) as well as other non-psychoanalytic approaches.

Behavioral activation (BA) is an evidence-based psychotherapy for depression based on the principle that decreased exposure to positive reinforcement leads to and maintains depressive symptoms. By systematically increasing engagement in meaningful or rewarding activities, BA aims to restore environmental reinforcement, reduce avoidance, and alleviate depression (Manos et al. 2010).

Of course, this was long before CBT existed as a method. At that time, it was not a competitor, so there were fewer reasons to reject it.

Bruno Walter (1876–1962) was a conductor, pianist, and composer. Born in Berlin, he left Germany in 1933 to escape the Third Reich, settling finally in the United States in 1939. He made recordings of significant historical and artistic significance and is widely considered one of the twentieth century's great conductors.

In 1906, Walter, then a young and ambitious conductor of great promise, consulted Sigmund Freud. Just when Walter had begun to enjoy the comforts of marriage and the economic security of a pleasant bourgeois existence, a "neurotic illness" struck him. He could no longer use his right arm for conducting or piano playing. *Theme and Variations: An Autobiography* (1946), Walter describes his encounter with Freud as follows:

> Instead of questioning me about sexual aberrations in infancy, as my layman's ignorance had led me to expect, *Freud examined my arm* briefly. I told him my story, feeling certain that he would be professionally interested in a possible connection between my actual physical affliction and wrong I had suffered more than a year before. Instead, he asked me if I had ever been to Sicily. When I replied that I had not, he said that it was very beautiful and interesting, and more Greek than Greece itself. In short, I was to leave that very evening, forget all about my arm and the Opera, and do nothing for a few weeks but use my eyes. I did as I was told … Mindful of Freud's instructions, I endeavored not to think of my affliction.

The trip to Sicily turned out to be a thrilling experience for Walter, but it did not heal his arm. Walter returned to Freud complaining about his pain:

I poured out my troubles to Freud. His advice was – to conduct.
"But I can't move my arm."
"Try it, at any rate.' '
And what if I should have to stop?' '
You won't have to stop.' '
Can I take upon myself the responsibility of possibly upsetting a
performance?"
"I'll take responsibility."

(pp. 164–168)

Freud offered Bruno Walter BA, and it helped. Many years later, it was yet formulated as one of the most widespread techniques within CBT. BA's goal is to increase environmental reinforcement and reduce punishment, and it sounds that this is precisely how it worked for Walter. Freud suggested two interventions: a vacation in Sicily, and when that did only partially, he insisted that Walter should conduct. He seems to have tried to reverse Walter's symptoms by telling him to engage in behavior that restores diverse and stable sources of positive reinforcement (the sheer pleasure of touring and looking at Sicily's sights) (Manos et al., 2010). He activated Walter and encouraged him to decrease avoidance and reengage in life in ways specific to Walter's values and goals and help Walter reestablish and sustain contact with positive reinforcement and prevent relapse.

Sterba (1951), who was intrigued by the therapeutic success of Freud's "simple, supportive method" (p. 78), interviewed Walter:

Bruno Walter had little to add in terms of a dynamic explanation of the treatment, but it was clear that he was still deeply impressed by Freud's personality forty-two years later. He stated that it was Freud's sincerity and decisiveness in his advice, which made him take the evening train to Genoa, the same day he had his first interview… The fact that Freud was able to take the responsibility that no upsetting of any performance would result from his trying to conduct again made him feel that he could try again and that he had to. In one of the following interviews, Freud asked him if in the state of being carried away by the music when he was conducting he did not sometimes forget about his ailment and conduct, using his right arm in an unhindered manner, which Bruno Walter had to confirm. And here Freud set in with further encouragement. He used this fact as a proof to the patient that he was able to overcome his neurotic affliction by conscious effort and encouraged him to continue doing just this. In a short time, Bruno Walter had overcome his neurosis. The whole treatment consisted of five to six interviews.

(pp. 78–79)

As mentioned, Walter became one of the foremost conductors of his times and never suffered a recurrence of his affliction. Sterba justly attributes the success of Freud's work to his depth assessment of Walter's psychodynamic equilibrium and his skill with which he used his suggestive authority. As Freud was prepared to assume full responsibility for a conducting failure, somehow, he inspired Walter's confidence that he could overcome his ailment on his own. Maybe Freud used here what Victor Frankl (1967) later called de-reflection.

By redirecting the attention or de-reflecting the attention away from the self, the person can become whole by thinking about others rather than themselves.

The fact that Freud did not publish the case, it could be argued, reflects that he did not consider it part of the psychoanalytic technique proper; thus, it ended up featuring as a treatment he did not bother to conceptualize. However, in other writings, Freud recommends using what we recognize now as CBT techniques with phobias.

Freud (1919) had stated that

> the various forms of disease treated by us cannot all be dealt with by the same technique. Our technique grew up in the treatment of hysteria and is still directed principally to the cure of that affection. But the phobias have already made it necessary for us to go beyond our former limits. One can hardly master a phobia if one waits till the patient lets the analysis influence him to give it up. He will never in that case bring into the analysis the material indispensable for a convincing resolution of the phobia. One must proceed differently. Take the example of agoraphobia; there are two classes of it, one mild, the other severe. Patients belonging to the first class suffer from anxiety when they go into the street by themselves, but they have not yet given up going out alone on that account; the others protect themselves from the anxiety by altogether ceasing to go about alone. With these last one succeeds only when one can induce them by the influence of the analysis to behave like phobic patients of the first class – that is, to go into the street and to struggle with their anxiety while they make an attempt. One starts, therefore, by moderating the phobia so far, and it is only when that has been achieved at the physician's demand that the associations and memories come into the patient's mind, which enable the phobia to be resolved.
>
> (pp. 165–166)

Indeed, Freud's theory included many ideas that could have served as the basis for the foundation of a psychoanalytic community supporting integrative therapy.

Javel (1999) pointed out that Beck's later discovery of automatic thoughts, which may have appeared novel, had already been anticipated in Freud's earlier writings, where he described similar phenomena that he termed involuntary thoughts. Accounting for his decision to replace the technique of hypnosis in favor of having the patient freely express their feelings and thoughts, Freud wrote that he had

> now found a substitute –and a completely satisfactory one – in the "associations" of the patients; that is, in the involuntary thoughts (most frequently regarded as disturbing elements and therefore ordinarily pushed aside) which so often break across the continuity of a consecutive narrative.
>
> (Freud, 1904/1958, p. 251)

In CBT, the uncovering of automatic thoughts leads the cognitive therapist to the patient's core beliefs, which are the assumptions underlying the patient's actions and reactions. Such core beliefs, once discovered, can be challenged and modified. Freud declares a similar objective: "The patient's symptoms and pathological manifestations, like all his mental processes, are of a very elaborately organized nature... Now we teach him to understand the structure of these highly complicated formations in his mind" (1919a/1958, p. 167).

Regarding technique, Freud writes, "[...] it would be possible for the pathogenic groups of ideas, that were after all certainly present, to be brought to life by mere insistence" (1895/1958, p. 268), much as the cognitive therapist "guides the patient to report her thoughts" (Beck, 1995, p. 88). Once the unconscious ideas and transference feelings are understood, Freud argues that there is more work to be done:

> We have been told that after the analysis of a sick mind a synthesis of it must follow.... But are we to leave it to the patient to deal alone with the resistances we have pointed out to him? Does it not seem natural that we should help him in another way, by putting him into the mental situation most favorable to solution of the conflict, which is our aim?... I think activity of such a kind on the part of the physician analyzing is unobjectionable and entirely justified.
>
> (1919/1958, pp. 159–162)

Such non-interpretive interventions, Freud calls "suggestion": "We take care of the patient's final independence by employing suggestion to get him to accomplish a piece of psychical work which has as its necessary result a permanent improvement in his psychical situation" (1912/1958, p. 106).

As if anticipating the rationale for integration, he writes, "In practice, it is true, that there is nothing to be said against a psychotherapist combining a certain amount of analysis with some suggestive influence to achieve a perceptible result in a shorter time" (Freud, 1919b/1958, p. 118). Freud does not elaborate on what suggestions to use. Still, based on the above quotations, we may conclude that using CBT techniques in some cases was naturally evident in some instances. Javel (1999) went so far as to claim that "classical psychoanalysis seems to be a divergent or 'dissenting' movement from Freud, and CBT seems to be a continuation" (p. 400).

Integrative thinking after Freud

Support for the idea of integration did not end with Freud's thinking. Other central actors in mainstream psychoanalysis were similarly supportive. Some called for integration directly and explicitly. Others supported a technique that was ostensibly psychoanalytically "pure" and yet incorporated elements of CBT.

Let us briefly examine some of these attempts.

More than 80 years ago, Thomas French wrote his article "Interrelations between Psychoanalysis and the Experimental Work of Pavlov" (1933). In this paper, French showed himself to be an early proponent of integrating different psychotherapies by comparing the psychoanalytic and Pavlovian conditioning approaches. Despite their differences, French thought that there were apparent similarities between the psychoanalytic idea of repression and the Pavlovian notion of extinction and inhibition. French attempted to find a link between sublimation and principles underpinning the process of learning by drawing attention to the principle of differentiation. He suggested that some form of discrimination training would probably enable an individual to tell the difference between what is socially acceptable or unacceptable of expressing specific drives. French also believed that earlier conditioning experiences are responsible for the ability to adjust to reality.

Taking French's ideas about integration a step further, Kubie (1934) argued that conditioned reflex might be a valuable concept for understanding psychoanalytic processes. Kubie thought that some meaningful associations remain outside of consciousness because they were acquired under a state of inhibition. He speculated that encouragement of a patient's free association and the relatively passive role adopted by the analyst might change original inhibition conditions, paving the way for earlier unconscious associations to become part of an individual's conscious awareness.

These early integrated psychotherapies were followed in 1950 by the landmark publication of Dollard and Miller's *Personality and Psychotherapy,* which they dedicated to "Freud and Pavlov and their students." The authors offered a detailed description of how psychoanalytic ideas such as regression, anxiety, repression, and displacement could be understood within the context of learning theory.

While Dollard and Miller remained relatively faithful to the techniques associated with classical psychoanalytic therapy, they repeatedly referred to principles and procedures which form the basis of the new behavioral treatment. For example, they stressed the importance of treatment of setting the patients a series of tasks to perform in a prearranged order of importance. The language they used was generally replete with the terminology of CBT, for instance: "[...] the therapist uses approval to reward good efforts on the part of the patient" (p. 395), or "[...] behavioral changes must be made in the real world of the patient's current life. If benevolent changes are to occur, the patient must begin doing something new" (p. 319).

Dollard and Miller also stressed the vital importance in the final therapy stages of teaching the patient how to exercise self-control or use his coping skills once the therapy has ended.

Alexander (1963), one of the most prominent leaders of mainstream psychoanalysis proposed that it may be of value to recordings of psychoanalytic therapy sessions, the patient learns a new interrelating pattern. This mainly unconscious learning conforms to Behaviorism's learning principles through positive reinforcement of a new and functional mode of interrelating.

Dedicated as he was to advancing the field throughout his career, Alexander believed he witnessed the start of integrating psychoanalytic theory and learning theory, which he hoped would lead to advances in all psychotherapies and approaches. Marmor (1964), involved in the same research on psychotherapy as Alexander, provided a detailed description of the learning principles, which, in his view, form the basis of psychoanalytic therapy.

Edward Glover's (1931) technique called "Neglect and Counter-Stimulation" (1931) also used behavioral methods. Glover was an orthodox and classical Freudian psychoanalyst (he vehemently opposed Melanie Klein due to his disloyalty to Freud's theory). But even he was tempted to borrow something from behavioral methods when he developed his "Neglect and Counter-Stimulation" method.

Glover believed that the use of "persuasive methods" in psychoanalysis could be beneficial. He thought that they belonged to a type of

> Inexact interpretation which, depending on an optimum degree of psychic remoteness from the true source of anxiety, may bring about improvement in the symptomatic sense at the cost of refractoriness to deeper analysis.
>
> (1931, p. 400)

> [...] the practitioner recommends his patient to embark on activities outside his customary routine. He advises a change of place (holiday) or of bodily habit (recreation, sport, etc.) or of mental activity (light reading, music-hall, etc.). The tendencies here are quite patent. The physician unwittingly tries to reinforce the mechanism of repression (neglect) and quite definitely invokes a system of counter-charge or anticathexis. His advice to go for a holiday or play golf or attend concerts is therefore, an incitement to substitute (symptom) formation. The physician encourages the patient by demonstrating his own capacity for repression. He says in effect, "You see, I am blind; I don't know what is the matter with you: go and be likewise".
>
> (p. 404)

Over the years, there was some interest in integration between psychoanalysis and CBT (Arkowitz & Messer, 1984; Connors, 2006; Shahar, 2010; Shahar & Govrin, 2017), but they were always sporadic and were not backed up by political organizations (On the history of integration, see Goldfried, 1982).

The psychologist most identified with the integration of psychodynamic and CBT is Paul Wachtel, whose *Psychoanalysis and Behavior Therapy Toward an Integration* was published in 1977 and became a classic.

Wachtel writes (1984):

> Arguments showing that psychoanalysis and behavior therapy are different do not really bear on the question of whether they can be integrated. Indeed, were they not rather different, there would be little point in an integration. The very fact that each stresses certain things that the other does not makes an integration more useful than either separately. And, of course, it is their differences that make an effort at integration interesting and challenging. It is no feat to put together what seems compatible and alike to everyone. As I conceive it, integration is not just a hodgepodge of eclecticism, a salad with a little of this and a little of that tossed in. The goal, rather, is the development of a new coherent structure, an internally consistent approach both to technical intervention and to the construction of theory.

An integrative or synthetic effort is built on both an admiring and a critical attitude toward each separate approach. It is admiring in the sense that each has something useful and important to contribute, and it is critical in the sense that each is seen as omitting something useful and important (for the most part, something that is part of what is valuable about the other approach.

(p. 45)

Since then, Wachtel wrote numerous papers and books on the subject (Wachtel, 2014, 2011). His theory of cyclical psychodynamics (Wachtel, 2014) is a version of relational thought that emphasizes how early patterns of interpersonal transaction and subjective experience are perpetuated in the present via vicious and virtuous circles; it integrates the components of CBT and learning theory. Wachtel, who defines himself as a relational analyst, found a home in the relational tradition that is more open to psychoanalysis influences from the outside world. However, even within the relational approach, he is almost the only one who represents integration.

Integrative Therapies: Success and Failure

As we have shown, there are good theoretical reasons to integrate active interventions, particularly CBT, into psychoanalytic treatment. Attempts to integrate are common within psychoanalysis. However, due to the psychoanalytic establishment's resistance, nothing has come of these. This failure does not represent the widespread use of integration between psychodynamic theories and CBT.

One of the key findings of a 2010 survey involving more than 2,000 therapists in North America (Cook et al., 2010) is that psychodynamic techniques (e.g., relate current problems to childhood and family experiences; help clients explore unconscious processes) are often used by practitioners. Indeed, one in three therapists used them with most of their clients, and a similar number used them with some of their clients. Such a high percentage of therapists use psychodynamic practices, including CBT practitioners, demonstrates that psychoanalytic methods are still widely used and of considerable value to many therapists. Therefore, integration of CBT and psychoanalysis is not merely a theoretical possibility: many practitioners apply it daily.

Indications of the Failure of Integration

Thus, initiatives by prominent figures like Kubie, Alexander, or French were like seeds planted in infertile soil, and so eventually, they withered. The various attempts ultimately failed to lead to further experiments, didn't arouse the community's curiosity, and were not evolved by other analysts. However, outside the psychoanalytic establishment, such integration was a huge success.

How do we determine that integration has failed? First, methods integrating CBT and psychoanalytic techniques are not taught *in psychoanalytic institutes*. The curriculum of the training programs in ten psychoanalytic institutes belonging to the American Psychoanalytic Association shows that not one of them included a course attempting to refer to CBT in psychoanalysis. (Some of these institutes do teach neuropsychoanalysis and research in infant observation.) Similarly, Adult Psychodynamic Psychotherapy Programs also lacked a course on CBT. One could assume that CBT might find a more easy entry into psychotherapy programs than traditional psychoanalytic training. But here, too, there was no reference to CBT.

Second, just a handful of papers on integrative therapies appear in psychoanalytic journals (Bambery et al., 2009; Frank, 1993; Gershy, 2017; Sacks, 2007).

Third, not one prominent psychoanalyst from the establishment – Melanie Klein, Heinz Kohuth, Wilfred Bion, Donald Winnicott, and Margaret Mahler – expressed interest in integration or raised the topic of CBT for debate. If the community's most influential and prominent voices showed no interest in integration, the community could hardly be expected to support it.

In brief, integration between CBT and psychoanalysis turned into a niche, an area of its own, prospering outside the psychoanalytic community. Those representing it became more identified with the integration movement than with the psychoanalytic establishment.

Reasons for the Failure of Integration

What then are the reasons for the failure? How can we explain the lack of a small community of analysts who follow Freud, Glover, Kubie, French, Alexander, and Wachtel that support integration? Why have neuropsychoanalysis and infant research become an integral part of psychoanalysis, forming two small independent communities, while integration with CBT has failed to do so?

I suggest five possible explanations for this lacuna.

Identity

As mentioned, professional identity, or self-definition, in every calling demands clear separation between it and other disciplines: any blurring of boundaries threatens the uniqueness of the profession. However, where boundaries are protected, there is always the risk of isolation and stagnation. Neuropsychoanalysis and infant research succeeded in forming communities because disciplines that do not directly compete with psychoanalysis are less threatening to its self-definition.

The Psychoanalytic Narrative

Every psychoanalytic approach has its narrative, a plot occurring over time. An infant develops, passing through significant stations in the first years of life; something in this process goes wrong and leads to psychopathology. Each psychoanalytic school – Freud, Klein, Bion, Kohut, and Kernberg – has its own narrative and uses it as a powerful tool in making sense of the patient.

Psychoanalytic narratives are astonishingly productive. They can create meaning for an almost infinite number of clinical phenomena. They are especially conducive for forging a hidden thematic link between the adult patient and her early experiences. By detecting themes, repeating behaviors, or reactions from the past in the present, the analyst finds causes for much of the patient's suffering. A solid and convincing narrative guides the analyst's attention and choice of interventions.

Psychoanalysts are indifferent to CBT because it is not an integral part of the main narrative; they use. It is regarded as an alien element in their internal coherency. Incorporating it will be strident, like including an unidentified flying object (UFO) in a Shakespeare play.

Accept or Reject All

Over and beyond the fact that psychoanalytical narratives do not welcome "foreign" elements that threaten their coherence, the theory itself – which generates the narratives – is a relatively closed system. That is to say, if you accept its therapeutic technique, you have to admit the system of assumptions on psychopathology, infant development, the nature of transference relations, and the perception of mental health on which that technique relies and to which it refers. It is difficult to accept some of the assumptions and not others. For therapeutic approaches that rely on a less complete and detailed view of human nature and psychopathology, it is, by contrast, more comfortable to borrow components from other therapeutic methods.

A Theory Under Siege

Psychoanalysis has been subject to harsh criticism for its lack of accessibility to empirical substantiation. In the past, the discipline did not address its therapeutic efficacy (something which over the past few years has changed substantially). Psychology journals publish only a few articles related to psychoanalysis. Psychoanalysts publish in their own journals, and their readership is limited to members of the psychoanalytic community. All this causes the psychoanalytic community to take a defensive position and further close itself to external influence.

Ignorance

Psychodynamic psychotherapists simply don't know enough about CBT. Their knowledge of it is anecdotal and superficial. Rice (2004), for example, who suggested a psychodynamic approach to obsessive-compulsive disorders, wrote:

> I personally have not seen patients who were treated with CBT nor am I competent to practice it, so I must defer to the literature and anecdotal information. However, though it may be of some help in reducing ritualistic behavior, I find it hard to imagine how it can positively affect obsessions.
>
> (p. 40)

Some Suggested Solutions

Expectations from the psychoanalytic community should be modest. If the Kleinian or adherents of self psychology, will make an effort to integrate components of CBT, this might adversely affect the coherence of their respective core theories and infringe on the identity of the community from which that theory crucially evolved (Govrin, 2015).

Single orientations communities dedicated to Bion, Klein, or Kohut should not be encouraged to incorporate nonanalytic components. Their devotion and research methods should be respected as well as their need for solid identity. Rather, a small community of organized analysts devoted to integration can serve as an important contribution. They should operate alongside the monolithic schools. Neuropsychoanalysis and infant research are exemplars for this kind of community. They do not replace the main theories of psychoanalysis but rather function as "sensibilities" (Govrin, 2019).

The rationale of such a community is that information afforded by CBT might, in some cases, contribute to the efficacy of specific treatments (Dimaggio & Lysaker, 2014). For example, when patients show certain symptoms, the therapy must focus on those and do it in a particular manner. As an illustration, a recent assessment contrasted psychodynamic therapy with CBT for eating disorders (Fairburn, 2008). In harmony with its worldview, psychodynamic therapists did not invite patients to explicitly concentrate on symptoms or assist them in overcoming problematic behaviors. Consistent with the dynamic approach, therapists did not initiate a discussion on eating habits. Results were remarkable: 20 sessions of CBT were higher than two years of psychodynamic therapy on any outcome measure.

From another perspective, Shedler (2012) indicates that the active ingredients of other therapies include unacknowledged psychodynamic elements. Shedler writes:

> Qualitative analysis of the verbatim session transcripts suggested that the poorer outcomes associated with cognitive interventions were due to implementation of the cognitive treatment model in dogmatic, rigidly insensitive ways by some of the therapists (Castonguay et al., 1996). (No school of therapy appears to have a monopoly on dogmatism or therapeutic insensitivity. Certainly, the history of psychoanalysis is replete with examples of dogmatic excesses.) On the other hand, the findings *do* indicate that the more effective therapists facilitated therapeutic processes that have long been core, centrally defining features of psychoanalytic theory and practice.
>
> (p. 104)

As Wachtel (2014) writes:

> Finding the right balance between openness to the value of others' work and belief in the value of one's own and one's confreres' is a delicate and continuous process, but it is an essential one, and hewing too close to either pole is likely to make real creativity unlikely.
>
> (p. 98)

One way for such a movement to arise is by adapting cognitive methods (Govrin, 2015) to better fit in with the psychoanalytic narrative in the same way as CBT did with mindfulness. If we calibrate CBT to match psychoanalysis' grand narrative, we may be more in a position to create a proud integrative community.

Here is a provisional and schematic outline for what such a project may look like:

a   A return to the sources shows that Freud and other significant psychoanalysis representatives used cognitive methods in their analytical work whenever they thought it might be effective.
b   Showing, by reference to already existing literature (e.g., Pilecki et al., 2015; Shedler, 2012), the areas of overlap between orthodox psychoanalytic theory and CBT.
c   Encouraging analysts to recognize CBT as being intrinsically linked to psychoanalysis by tracing CBT's wide range of techniques in psychoanalytic thought.

Conclusion

The history traced in this chapter reveals a paradox at the heart of psychoanalysis: a discipline founded on the exploration of resistance has itself become remarkably resistant to certain forms of influence. What makes this resistance particularly striking is not merely that it exists, but that it persists despite compelling internal logic for integration. Freud himself demonstrated that cognitive and behavioral interventions could serve psychoanalytic goals; prominent figures within the establishment repeatedly gestured toward synthesis; and yet no sustainable community of integrative practice took root within mainstream psychoanalysis.

This failure speaks to something deeper than theoretical incompatibility or empirical disagreement. The five barriers identified here—identity threat, narrative coherence, systemic wholeness, defensive posture, and simple ignorance—ultimately converge on a single underlying dynamic: the profound difficulty of encountering otherness without experiencing it as a challenge to one's professional existence. When neuropsychoanalysis and infant research succeeded where CBT integration failed, it was not because they offered superior insights, but because they posed no direct threat to psychoanalysis's self-conception as a distinct method of treatment. They enriched psychoanalytic theory without competing for its therapeutic soul.

Yet acknowledging this failure need not lead to resignation. The barriers documented here point toward philosophical questions that demand more sophisticated frameworks than have typically been brought to bear on therapeutic integration. How can one genuinely welcome foreign ideas without losing theoretical coherence? What does it mean for approaches to influence each other when they operate from fundamentally different premises about human nature and change? Can theoretical development proceed through processes more complex than conscious borrowing or defensive rejection? The chapters that follow take up these questions not as abstract puzzles but as lived challenges confronting anyone who seeks to think seriously about therapeutic encounter across difference.

What emerges across this volume is not a blueprint for dissolving psychoanalysis into eclecticism, nor a manifesto for protecting it from contamination. Rather, we develop philosophical resources for understanding integration as a more nuanced phenomenon than either wholesale adoption or rigid exclusion. The modest proposal advanced here—for a small integrative community operating alongside monolithic schools—anticipates this richer account. It recognizes that meaningful encounter with otherness requires both spaces of protection (where theoretical traditions can develop their internal logic without constant defensive posturing) and spaces of experimentation (where practitioners can risk crossing borders without abandoning their intellectual homes). The future of therapeutic integration may depend less on converting the resistant than on creating conditions where different forms of engagement with difference can coexist, each contributing to a more vibrant ecology of therapeutic thought and practice.

References

Alexander, F. (1963). The dynamics of psychotherapy in light of learning theory. *American Journal of Psychiatry, 120*, 440–448.

Arkowitz, H., & Messer, S. B. (Eds.). (1984). *Psychoanalytic therapy and behavior therapy: Is integration possible?* New York: Plenum Press.

Bambery, M., Porcerelli, J. H., & Ablon, J. S. (2009). Prototypes of psychodynamic and CBT psychotherapy with adolescents: Development and applications for training. *Journal of the American Psychoanalytic Association, 57*(1), 175–181. https://doi.org/10.1177/0003065108331278

Beck, J. S. (1995). *Cognitive therapy: Basics and beyond.* New York: Guilford Press.

Blass, R. B., & Carmeli, Z. (2007). The case against neuropsychoanalysis: On fallacies underlying psychoanalysis' latest scientific trend and its negative impact on psychoanalytic discourse. *The International Journal of Psychoanalysis, 88*(1), 19–40. https://doi.org/10.1516/6NCA-A4MA-MFQ7-0JTJ

Bornstein, R. F. (2001). The impending death of psychoanalysis. *Psychoanalytic Psychology, 18*(1), 3–20. https://doi.org/10.1037/0736-9735.18.1.2

Castonguay, L. G., Goldfried, M. R., Wiser, S. L., Raue, P. J., & Hayes, A. M. (1996). Predicting the effect of cognitive therapy for depression: A study of unique and common factors. *Journal of Consulting and Clinical Psychology, 64*, 497–504. https://psycnet.apa.org/doi/10.1037/0022-006X.64.3.497

Connors, M. E. (2006). *Symptom-Focused dynamic psychotherapy.* Mahwah, NJ: Analytic Press.

Cook, J. M., Biyanova, T., Elhai, J., Schnurr, P. P., & Coyne, J. C. (2010). What do psychotherapists really do in practice? An Internet study of over 2,000 practitioners. *Psychotherapy: Theory, Research, Practice, Training, 47*(2), 260–267. https://doi.org/10.1037/a0019788

David, D. (2014). Some concerns about the psychological implications of mindfulness: A critical analysis. *Journal of Rational-Emotive & Cognitive-Behavior Therapy, 32*(4), 313–324. https://doi.org/10.1007/s10942-014-0198-z

Dimaggio, G., & Lysaker, P. H. (2014). Supporters of a single orientation may do less for science and the health of patients than integrationists: A reply to Govrin (2014). *Journal of Psychotherapy Integration, 24*(2), 91–94. https://psycnet.apa.org/doi/10.1037/a0036996

Dollard, J., & Miller, N. E. (1950). *Personality and psychotherapy; an analysis in terms of learning, thinking, and culture.* New York: McGraw-Hill.

Fairburn, C. G. (Ed.). (2008). *Cognitive behavior therapy and eating disorders.* New York: Guilford Press.

Frank, K. A. (1993). Action, insight, and working through: Outline of an integrative approach. *Psychoanalytic Dialogues, 3*(4), 535–577. https://doi.org/10.1080/10481889309538993

Frankl, V. E. (1967). *The doctor and the soul: From psychotherapy to logotherapy* (Rev. ed., pp. 208–209). New York: Vintage Books

French, T. M. (1933). Interrelations between psychoanalysis and the experimental work of Pavlov. *The American Journal of Psychiatry, 12,* 1165–1203. https://doi.org/10.1176/ajp.89.6.1165

Freud, S. (1919). Lines of advance in psychoanalytic therapy. In J. Strachey (Ed. and Trans.), *The standard edition of the complete psychological works of Sigmund Freud.* S.E., 17 London: Hogarth Press.

Freud, S. (1895/1958). The psychotherapy of hysteria. In J. Strachey (Ed. and Trans.), *The standard edition of the complete psychological works of Sigmund Freud* (Vol. 2, p. 268). London: Hogarth Press.

Freud, S. (1904/1958). Freud's psychoanalytic procedure. In J. Strachey (Ed. and Trans.), *The standard edition of the complete psychological works of Sigmund Freud* (Vol. 7, p. 251). London: Hogarth Press.

Freud, S. (1912/1958). The dynamics of transference. In J. Strachey (Ed. and Trans.), *The standard edition of the complete psychological works of Sigmund Freud* (Vol. 12, p. 106). London: Hogarth Press.

Freud, S. (1919/1958a). Lines of advance in psychoanalytic therapy. In J. Strachey (Ed. and Trans.), *The standard edition of the complete psychological works of Sigmund Freud* (Vol. 17, pp. 159–162, 167). London: Hogarth Press.

Freud, S. (1919/1958b). Recommendations to physicians practicing psychoanalysis. In J. Strachey (Ed. and Trans.), *The standard edition of the complete psychological works of Sigmund Freud* (Vol. 17, p. 118). London: Hogarth Press.

Gershy, N. (2017). Psychodynamic case formulation: A roadmap to protocol adaptation in CBT. *Psychoanalytic Psychology, 34*(4), 478–487. https://doi.org/10.1037/pap0000104

Glover, E. (1931). The therapeutic effect of inexact interpretation: A contribution to the theory of suggestion. *The International Journal of Psychoanalysis, 12,* 397–411

Goldfried, M. R. (1982). On the history of therapeutic integration. *Behavior Therapy, 13*(5), 572–593. https://dx. doi.org/10.1016/S0005-7894(82)80017-8

Govrin, A. (2015). *Relational perspectives book series: Vol. 72. Conservative and radical perspectives on psychoanalytic knowledge: The fascinated and the disenchanted.* Routledge: Taylor & Francis Group.

Govrin, A. (2019). Facts and sensibilities: What is a psychoanalytic innovation? *Frontiers in Psychology, 10,* 1781. https://doi.org/10.3389/fpsyg.2019.01781

Green, A. (2000). Science and science fiction in infant research. In J. Sandler, A.- M. Sandler, & R. Davies (Eds.), *Clinical and observational psychoanalytic research: Roots of a controversy* (pp. 41–72). Madison, CT: International Universities Press.

Harman, O., & Diertrich, R. D. (2013). *Outsider scientists -routes to innovation in biology.* Chicago: Chicago University Press.

Harrington, N., & Pickles, C. (2009). Mindfulness and cognitive behavioral therapy: Are they compatible concepts? *Journal of Cognitive Psychotherapy, 23*, 315–323. https://doi.org/10.1891/0889-8391.23.4.315

Hayes, S. C., & Hofmann, S. G. (2017). The third wave of cognitive behavioral therapy and the rise of process-based care. *World Psychiatry, 16*(3), 245–246. https://doi.org/10.1002/wps.20442

Hofmann, S. G., & Asmundson, G. J. G. (2008). Acceptance and mindfulness-based therapy: New wave or old hat? *Clinical Psychology Review, 28*, 1–16. https://doi.org/10.1016/j.cpr.2007.09.003

Javel, A. F. (1999). The Freudian antecedents of cognitive-behavioral therapy. *Journal of Psychotherapy Integration, 9*(4), 397–407.

Kohut, H. (1978). *The search for the self, volume 2: Selected writings of Heinz Kohut 1950–1978.* New York: International University Press.

Kubie, L. S. (1934). Body symbolization and the development of language. *Psychoanalytic Quarterly, 3*, 430–444.

Lakatos, I. (1978). *The methodology of scientific research programmes.* Cambridge: Cambridge University Press.

Leahy, R. L. (2008). A closer look at ACT. *The Behavior Therapist, 31*, 148–150.

Levenson, T. (2015). *The hunt for Vulcan.* New York: Random House.

Laudan, L., Donovan, A., Laudan, R., Barker, P., Brown, H., Leplin, J., Thagrad, P., & Wyksrea, S. (1986). Scientific change: Philosophical models and historical (Vol. 69, No. 2), Testing Theories of Scientific Change (Nov., 1986), pp. 141–223 Published by: Springer. URL: https://www.jstor.org/stable/20116337 Accessed: 02/09/2009, 05:14.

Manos, R. C., Kanter, J. W., & Busch, A. M. (2010). A critical review of assessment strategies to measure the behavioral activation model of depression. *Clinical Psychology Review, 30*(5), 547–561. https://doi.org/10.1016/j.cpr.2010.03.008

Marmor, J. (1964). Psychoanalytic therapy and theories of learning. In Masserman, J. (Ed), *Science and psychoanalysis* (Vol. 7). New York: Grune & Stratton.

Musser, G. (2016). *Spooky action at a distance: The phenomenon that reimagines space and time--and what it means for Black Holes, the Big Bang, and theories of everything.* New York: Farrar Straus and Giroux.

Pilecki, B., Thoma, N., & McKay, D. (2015). Cognitive behavioral and psychodynamic therapies: Points of intersection and divergence. *Psychodynamic Psychiatry, 43*(4), 463–490.

Rice, E. (2004). Reflections on the obsessive-compulsive disorders: A psychodynamic and therapeutic perspective. *Psychoanalytic Review, 91*(1), 23–44. https://doi.org/10.1521/prev.91.1.23.33826

Rustin, J. (2013). *Infant research and neuropsychoanalysis at work in psychotherapy: Expanding the clinical repertoire.* New York: Norton.

Sacks, M. (2007). BI-LOGIC as a bridge between psychoanalysis and CT and as a theoretical rationale for Beck's cognitive distortions. *British Journal of Psychotherapy, 23*(3), 383–394.

Seligman, S. (2018). *Relationships in development: Infancy, intersubjectivity, and attachment.* New York: Routledge.

Shahar, G. (2010). Poetics, pragmatics, schematics, and the psychoanalysis-research dialogue (Rift). *Psychoanalytic Psychotherapy, 24*(4), 315–328. https://doi.org/10.1080/02668734.2010.513544

Shahar, G., & Govrin, A. (2017). Psychodynamizing and existentializing cognitive–behavioral interventions: The case of behavioral activation (BA). *Psychotherapy, 54*(3), 267–272. https://doi.org/10.1037/pst0000115

Shedler, J. (2012). *The efficacy of psychodynamic psychotherapy.* In R. A. Levy, J. S. Ablon, & H. Kächele (Eds.), *Psychodynamic psychotherapy research: Evidence-based practice and practice-based evidence* (pp. 9–25). Heidelberg: Humana Press, Springer Nature. https://doi.org/10.1007/978-1-60761-792-1_2

Sterba, R. (1951). A case of brief psychotherapy by Sigmund Freud. *Psychoanalytic Review, 38*(1), 75–80.

Stern, D. N. (2010). *Forms of vitality: Exploring dynamics experience in psychology, the arts, psychotherapy and development.* Oxford: Oxford University Press.

Walter, B. (1946). *Theme and variations: An autobiography.* New York: Alfred A. Knopf.

Wachtel, P. L. (1984). *Psychoanalysis and behavior therapy: Toward an integration.* Basic Books.

Wachtel, P. L. (2011). *Inside the session: What really happens in psychotherapy.* American Psychological Association.

Wachtel, P. L. (2014). *Cyclical psychodynamics and the contextual self: The inner world, the intimate world, and the world of culture and society.* Routledge.

Wootton, D. (2016). *The invention of science: A new history of the scientific revolution.* London: Penguin.

Yovell, Y., Solms, M., & Fotopoulou, A. (2015). The case for neuropsychoanalysis: Why a dialogue with neuroscience is necessary but not sufficient for psychoanalysis. *The International Journal of Psychoanalysis, 96*(6), 1515–1553. https://doi.org/10.1111/1745-8315.12332

Psychoanalysis and CBT

From Rivalry to Hospitality in Psychotherapy Integration

Yael Peri Herzovich and Aner Govrin

Throughout this chapter, we will see that despite the many efforts to integrate psychoanalysis with cognitive-behavioral therapy (CBT), many loyal therapists of each school have consistently refused to "open their gate" to the other's influence. We explain this resistance as a way to reserve a strong professional identity through the us-them distinction. Any attempt to encourage loyal therapists to be influenced by the other school must guarantee that the other will not threaten their identity. We use Derrida's notion of hospitality to facilitate mutual influence between the schools while overcoming the other's threatening encounter. According to Derrida, hospitality, in response to the law of ethics, opens the home's threshold to the foreigner; in this law, the other is always welcome. At the same time, hospitality prevents a hostile takeover – by the law of politics, which ensures the owner's ongoing control over his house. By thus keeping the tension between openness and control over who enters, hospitality makes listening and learning between the psychotherapeutic schools possible. We discuss practical ways to put the concept of hospitality to work between the two schools, offer illustrations, and argue for this model's advantages.

The Struggle Between the Schools

Sigmund Freud and Aaron Beck, the founding fathers of psychoanalysis and CBT, were both open to incorporating "foreign" therapeutic elements when they worked with their patients. Freud (1919) recommended using behavioral techniques with phobic patients, and Beck developed a theory of dreams that he presented to both psychoanalysts and behavior therapists (Rosner, 2002). However, their loyal followers failed to show the same open-minded stance. The history of both movements has been marked by each school's way of asserting itself through bitter antagonism and competition with the other school (Norcross & Alexander, 2019). Indeed, each school of thought represents a different and even clashing cultural tradition, understanding human suffering, the mind, therapeutic objectives, practices, and change processes.

The two schools consist of a cluster of theories and therapeutic methods, each of which again includes tendencies that are variously at odds. Here we will refer

DOI: 10.4324/9781003608103-3

to their respective most central and mainstream approach (Blagys & Hilsenroth, 2000, 2002; Gardner, 2017; Milton, 2001).

The classic cognitive-behavioral approach, which rests mainly on Beck's (1976) and Ellis's (1962) cognitive models and early theories of learning (Skinner, 1953; Wolpe, 1969) and the classical psychodynamic approach, based on the principles of psychoanalysis theoretically formulated by Freud (1913), reflect profoundly different world views. While behavioral psychotherapists tend to have a realist, objective, and extrospective orientation, psychodynamic therapists' orientation is inclined to the idealist, subjective, and introspective. These divergent perspectives yield divergent basic assumptions regarding the nature of reality and human possibilities and constraints. Psychoanalytic theory is marked by a romantic outlook (driven by struggle and conflict), ironic (focused on inner contradiction, vagueness, and paradox), and tragic (underlining danger, terror, and the absurdity of human existence). It directs toward reflection and investigation. By contrast, the CBT has more in common with a comic view of the world (emphasizing the familiar, predictable, and controllable in humans and social situations). It expresses itself in action (Kubacki & Chase, 1998; Messer & Winokur, 1980).

Adherents of the psychodynamic approach argue that the cognitive-behavioral approach, relying on a narrow notion of the human condition, focuses on learning and information processing processes and fails to register humans' position on a crossroads of historical, developmental, and cultural continuums. Hence, wherever problems are complex, the approach is limited (Milton, 2001; Shahar, 2011a). As concerns those subscribing to the cognitive-behavioral model, they consider psychodynamic interpretations as an illusion of understanding at the expense of clarity, precision, and the predictive ability offered by behavioral assessments and interventions (Lewis, 1970). Their main argument is that psychotherapy, as they see it, should be a scientifically confirmed, evidence-based approach that can be proven effective (Marom, 2010). Evidence shows support for CBT's efficacy for a wide range of psychiatric disorders (Butler et al., 2006; Hofmann & Smits, 2017).

For many years, psychotherapists believed that CBT enjoys a superior standing in terms of evidence-based research, and by contrast, that psychodynamic therapies are not scientifically validated. However, this conclusion has proven to be wrong. Many studies have validated psychodynamic treatments' efficacy in a wide range of psychiatric disorders in the last decade. Studies have consistently demonstrated that psychodynamic therapy benefits not only endure over time but also increase with time (Leichsenring et al., 2015; Leuzinger-Bohleber et al., 2003; Shedler, 2010; Steinert et al., 2017).

Furthermore, representatives of the psychodynamic approach, like Westen, Novotny, and Thompson-Brenner (2004), have argued that cognitive-behavioral researchers ignored specific details, set aside evidence, or even presented false evidence. Shedler (2015), CBT's most vehement opponent, has argued that CBT's research practices paint a misleading picture of the actual benefits of "evidence-based" therapies, including sham control groups, cherry-picked patient samples, and suppression of negative findings. Furthermore, he claimed that empirical research shows that "evidence-based" therapies are ineffective treatments and their benefits are trivial. Few patients get well, and even the trivial benefits do not last. Crits-Christoph, Wilson, and Hollon (2005), defending these studies and belonging to the other camp, argued that Westen and colleagues are entirely incorrect in their claims; that randomized controlled trials remain the most powerful way to test notions of causal agency. Edelstein, Kujoth, and Ramsay Steele (2013), also representatives of the cognitive-behavioral approach, argue that the psychodynamic method is archaic and superannuated, and should only make its appearance on the TV or cinema screens.

Over time, the schools' divisions were so great that there was no opportunity for a genuine dialogue. Instead of being a platform for rendezvous and exchanging knowledge, scientific research became another arena for the struggle over control. This antagonism escalated and turned contemptuous and dismissive, rather than maintaining a dispassionate academic tone.

Although both forms of psychotherapy proved their efficacy, the battle is far from being over. Indeed, some of the scientific attention shifted to study the effectiveness of each approach by types of disorders, while another direction shifted from outcome-focused research to process-focused research on common factors and specific ingredients (Wampold & Ulvenes, 2019). But despite significant progress, little consensus has been reached. Critical questions that go beyond statistics like choosing the best therapy for a specific patient to treat a particular problem are not considered among each school's loyal therapists. It seems that "no school of therapy appears to have a monopoly on dogmatism or therapeutic insensitivity" (Shedler, 2010, p. 104).

The battle also involves economic competition over public resources, recognition, and prestige (Milton, 2001; Shahar, 2011b). The contest influences processes of study, training, and specialization. Political, social, and economic forces, like professional organizations and training institutions, continue to hold individuals tethered to a single approach, which causes them to avoid the contributions of alternative orientations (Norcross & Alexander, 2019).

Attempts to Bring the Schools Closer

Before the schools were established as rival schools, many psychoanalysts felt free to use behavioral techniques. Freud used behavioral techniques with some of his patients (e.g., the famous composer Bruno Walter; Walter, 1946). Hardcore psychoanalysts like Lawrence Kubie (1934) and Edward Glover (1931) also used similar CBT techniques. Aaron Beck, who began his professional way as a psychoanalytic researcher, emphasized the similarities between CBT and the psychodynamic approach (Rosner, 2012).

During the last decades, the integration movement in psychotherapy has presented the initial attempt to overcome the schools' conflict (Arkowitz & Messer, 1984; Goldfried, Pachankis & Goodwin, 2019; Messer, 1986; Norcross & Alexander, 2019). The assumption is that no single approach can address all challenges in one domain: there are overlaps between the tendencies, and their combined use might significantly add to psychotherapeutic effectiveness (Ziv-Beiman & Shahar, 2014).

Still, the two schools' respective training programmes, conferences, and influential journals hardly mention other perspectives. Each school's loyal followers continue to ignore each other's existence, oblivious to any possible integration. This fact contrasts with the astounding number of clinicians who refuse to identify with a one-school approach and use more than one therapeutic orientation (Cook et al., 2010).

How can we explain the contempt and animosity that characterize the loyal followers of each group? Loyal therapists from one camp perceive other therapists as strangers who might pose a threat to their worldview. "What lies outside might be not only not noticed but actively rejected since it is associated with a point of view that is derided and disdained as 'other'," in Wachtel's words (2010, p. 407). Wachtel (2010, 2018) sees the field of psychotherapy as divided between "tribal organizations" entangled in a culture war, something more like an ethnic conflict with its attendant us-versus-them feelings than an intellectual or scientific discussion. Differences are polarized; caricature and stereotype abound; each side is intensely attached to its own way, and self-definition is achieved by diminishing the other.

The similarity between the ethnic divide and psychotherapeutic communities' rivalry is significant. It means that the main obstacle to openness between the two schools is maintaining the us-them distinction and emphasizing salient differences to sustain professional-cultural identity. The group needs to hold convictions about what it believes and what it rejects for a stable and robust identity. The other group is used to strengthen one's group identity by putting this group outside the wall. As a result, mental barriers are formed which keep out the threat and keep the subject at a safe intellectual distance. Crossing the border to start a dialogue of some sort is perceived as threatening one's own identity.

Therefore, under these conditions, the question we pose is, what can help reduce this threat and enable an encounter and mutual influence between the two rival psychotherapeutic schools without endangering their identities?

Pragmatism and Theoretical Pluralism

Surprisingly, the integrative literature has paid little attention to what might facilitate the encounter with the other. Even when it discussed the role of communicating with the other (Safran & Messer, 1997; Stricker, 2010; Wachtel, 2010), the literature did not offer ways to overcome the identity threat.

The two main rationales to justify integration are pragmatic truth and theoretical pluralism. Regarding pragmatism, therapists should be looking for the best and most effective methods to help alleviate their patients' suffering. Integrating approaches make sense since both therapies were found to be effective (Gardner, 2017; Laska, Gurman & Wampold, 2014). But the widespread argument among integrationists that integration is "effective for the patient" or that it has been scientifically proven fails to convince either side of the debate that a sincere encounter and mutual open-mindedness are worth a try. Since each of them has different ideas about what can count as an effective therapy, they are often impenetrable to research evidence (Wachtel, 2018).

Integrationists' second rationale comes in the form of theoretical pluralism, according to which there is not one uniform means of approaching truths about the world, but rather many. The integration movement endorses the pluralist psychotherapeutic theory (Safran & Messer, 1997), psychotherapeutic practice (Downing, 2004), research (Anchin, 2008), and even ethics (Mahoney, 2005). The aim here is for further open-mindedness and exposure to alternative models. However, such an epistemological argument does not seem to be enough because no matter how right and politically correct, advancing pluralism remains external to the profession. Rather than aspiring to pluralism, loyal therapists of each school want to benefit their patients by sticking to their own principles. After all, why would foreign approaches influence therapists if they are convinced that their own system is the most effective one?

Since pragmatism and pluralism fail to convince loyal therapists to be open to other schools, we have to take a different turn and consult the rich philosophical literature concerning the encounter with the other. In this chapter, we propose one way of achieving an open-minded stance between loyal followers of each school by looking at Jacques Derrida's hospitality notion. Derrida's hospitality suggests a new perspective on communication between schools and between establishments and training institutes. It holds out a new way of refining our thinking on the subject and cast a new light on integrating the two schools.

On Hospitality

What Is Hospitality?

The Cambridge Dictionary definition of the word "hospitality" defines it as an act of being friendly and welcoming to guests and visitors. But Derrida offers a more intricate and nuanced understanding of this concept. In dialogue with Levinas's writings (Levinas, 1961, 1974), Derrida evolved his notion of hospitality (Derrida, 1991,1997a, 1997b, 1999, 2000, 2001, 2004, 2005). For Levinas, the very essence of language is friendship and hospitality. Hospitality is a fundamentally discursive phenomenon, directed at the other or the face of the other. Drawing out the link between hospitality and Levinas's acceptance of the face of the other, Derrida argues that orientation and attention toward speech, receptivity, and hospitality are the same thing (1997a). Hospitality, for him, signifies receiving the other, the stranger, into my home: "What 'hospitality' is and means, namely, to 'welcome,' 'accept,' 'invite,' 'receive,' 'bid,' someone welcome 'to one's home,' wherein one's own home, one is master of the household" (Derrida, 2000, p. 6).

The notion of hospitality touches on the relations between the same and the different, crossing boundaries, and negotiations between inside and outside. Rather than to friends and relatives, the question of hospitality directs itself to members of another group, another culture. As part of his social and political argument, Derrida deploys the notion, in the postcolonial, post-World War II discussion on the foreigner (Still, 2010). Nevertheless, the stranger's question is also an all-encompassing one, referring to all who are not me, outside the boundaries of my culture and language.

Therefore, one way of defining the stranger is in terms of language: She or he is foreign to the language in which hospitality occurs and how its rules are formulated (Derrida, 1997b). The language in which the stranger is listened to – should there be a willingness to do so, "is the ensemble of culture, it is the values, the norms, the meanings that inhabit the language. Speaking the same language is not only a linguistic operation. It's a matter of ethos generally" (1997b, p. 133). The definition of the stranger, in other words, refers to language qua culture and culture as hospitality.

For Derrida, hospitality, over and beyond being a potential encounter between cultural groups, between self and other, is the very essence of culture. It is not merely an ethical value but ethics itself (Derrida, 2001). But in his deconstructive analysis of the notion, he argues that the ethics of hospitality limits and contradicts itself from the outset. This results from the aporetic nature of the twofold law of hospitality, including the law of ethics and politics' laws with their tense and complex interrelations.

The law of ethics is unconditional. Under its regime, otherness is never put to the test, the other is not asked for her or his identity, acceptance is absolute, and they are always welcome. The other under this law constitutes a transcendental demand – a reflection of Levinas's influence on Derrida's thinking (Schoenfeld, 2007):

> Absolute hospitality requires that I open up my home and that I give not only to the foreigner (provided with a family name, with the social status of being a foreigner, etc.), but to the absolute, unknown, anonymous other, and that I give place to them, that I let them come, that I let them arrive, and take place in the place I offer them, without asking of them either reciprocity (entering into a pact) or even their names (Derrida, 1997b, p. 25).

The political law clashes with this unconditional ethical law. It is conditional, draws boundaries, is selective about its guests, examines passers-by, and demands they identify themselves before entering the home: it determines who is invited, thus defining the laws of hospitality (Schoenfeld, 2007). "Conditional hospitality where one invites, accepts, asks the name, imposes conditions, requires a visa: Come into my home, my country, but careful, specific rules must be respected" (Derrida, 2004, p. 49).

The need for the law of politics arises because the proprietor of the home must remain in charge of the home so that she or he does not turn from a host into hostage. The ethical law of absolute, unconditional hospitality pushes against the political law of respecting boundaries; the political law, in its turn, infringes the unconditional ethical law. At the same time, conditional laws take their inspiration from the unconditional law of hospitality. And while ethical law is superior to all other laws, it also needs them. To be what it is, it lays its formative claim on them, for they are what makes hospitality concretely possible. This is the antinomy (a fundamental and unresolvable contradiction) and aporia (a logical impasse) that Derrida explores – a contradiction that cannot be resolved or reduced between the two law regimes; they exclude each other, but at the same time they are bound and necessary to each other.

Hospitality and Hostility

Derrida points out the common Latin origin and root of the words "hospitality" and "hostility," "hostis as host and hostis as an enemy" (2000, p. 15) to further elaborate the antinomy and aporia of the double law of hospitality and how the concept includes its inverse. Every act of hospitality consists of a tension between invitation [of the guest] and hostility [toward the enemy]. Thus, it carries the traces of the violent nature from which it chooses to disconnect itself. On the one hand, the law of ethics demands: "fraternity, humanity, hospitality: the welcome of the other or the face as a neighbor and as a stranger, as neighbor insofar as he is a stranger, man and brother" (Derrida, 1997a, p. 68). Yet the conditional laws, right from the start, while protecting both host and guest against violence, are instruments of violence themselves. First, the host is the sovereign and the one in power; he decides to whom he grants hospitality, which requires exclusion. Second, since hospitality occurs within language or discourse, it always seeks to understand something about the guest in its terms, imposing itself on the other whom it hosts. Third, the host sets the hospitality rules and imposes them on the guest to make sure he maintains his identity and boundaries and stays in charge of his own home. And finally, hospitality depends on the guest giving something in return in gratitude for the extended hospitality:

> The host remains the master in the house, the country, the nation, he controls the threshold, controls the borders, and welcomes the guest he wants to keep the mastery. "I am the master of the house, the city, the nation" – that is what is implied in this form of conditional hospitality (Derrida, 1999, p. 69).

Derrida's notion of hospitality describes the encounter with the other and its inherent tension between openness to inviting the other and the boundaries' violent protection.

Hospitality is always about answering for a dwelling place, for one's identity, space, and limits, for the ethos as home (Derrida, 1997b). By crossing the home's threshold, the stranger casts doubt and unsettles the master's dogmas. And just like the host's identity and ethos come under threat, the other, foreigner whose invitation is conditional on specific conditions and obligations, faces a threat from the moment he crosses the threshold.

Why then should we host and be guests despite these threats? What do both host and guests can expect to gain when both identity and ethos will be challenged?

Derrida's (1997b) answer is that the question posed by the hospitality of the foreigner amounts to an invitation to the host to enter his own home (for Derrida, every concept includes its opposite; in French, the word *hôte* refers to both host and guest), and that the stranger may serve to liberate the master:

> The stranger could save the master and liberate the power of his host; it's as if the master, qua master, were a prisoner of his place and his power, of his ipseity, of his subjectivity (his subjectivity is hostage). So it is indeed the master, the one who invites, the inviting host, who becomes the hostage – and who always has been. And the guest, the invited hostage, becomes the one who invites the one who invites, the master of the host. The guest becomes the host's host (1997b, pp. 123–5).

And so, the host, convinced he is master of the house, is the recipient of the hospitality he offers within his home. His being host to his own hospitality sets him free of the alienation he experiences within his own home and situates him in it. While the stranger's question brings the risk of compromising the home's stability, it might also contribute to the answer, confirm its boundaries, and help them emerge clearly for all to see. This offers an opportunity to expand the limits of the answer, and thus to extend the home. Both guests and hosts must take the risk of hospitality for these gains to materialize.

Hospitality within the psychotherapeutic milieu

The concept of hospitality opens new possibilities for a new stance of openness between different schools in psychotherapy. The space we have in mind is, of course, intellectual rather than physical. But here, too, clearly articulated boundaries exist. Here again, there are members of the household and intruders. We can ask, right from the outset, why in the field of psychotherapy, the notion of hospitality is not particularly common. The representatives of the two schools, it seems, do not think of themselves as hosting the other side in their home territory. Usually, the feeling is that the encounter takes place on the battlefield. The respective representatives feel they must stake it out and fence it off to prevent a hostile takeover. The engagement takes place, for example, on the pages of professional journals or at mental health institutions: no man's land in which neither one of the tendencies usually predominates. It happens very rarely that one approach invites the other into its home. For example, it is rare to witness psychotherapists from one school lecture in the other school's training[1] programs.

We believe that the notion of hospitality introduces a new and radical direction for developing a new mental position among the most diehard supporters of each of these schools. To make this argument, we shall explore the notion of hospitality: Why is it worthwhile? How and under what circumstances can it be achieved? How might it be applied?

Why? – The Motivation for Hospitality

Questions about the motivation for hospitality touch upon the potential contribution and gains for the opposing parties involved. What motivates bringing the two approaches together is more than anything an awareness for each of them of incompleteness on their own. Here the believers, despite the great esteem in which they hold the method they work with, can see that it lacks something and that something coming from outside may help reduce that lack (Govrin, 2015, pp. 50–5). Indeed, many theoreticians and studies in each school have found that these approaches, when followed exclusively, are insufficient and partial (Castonguay, Newman & Holtforth, 2019; Jones & Pulos, 1993; Stricker & Gold, 2019; Zilcha-Mano & Errázuriz, 2015). Thus, for reasons of effectiveness, they constitute motivation for integration. However, as we already noted, evidence-based studies that point to effectiveness do not persuade the schools' loyalists to welcome foreign ideas.

Derrida's elaboration of welcoming the other offers a promising way to understand what each side can gain from a new encounter. For Derrida, the stranger does not merely constitute a threat to the cultural community's self-identity: it equally functions as what allows this identity to emerge. After all, self-constitution always occurs in the face of the other:

> The singularity of the "who" is not the individuality of a thing that would be identical to itself; it's not an atom. It is a singularity which dislocates or divides itself in gathering itself together to answer to the other, whose call somehow precedes its own identification with itself, for to this call I can only answer, have already answered, even if I think I am answering "no" (Derrida, 1991, p. 6).

Hence, both psychotherapeutic schools constitute themselves as separate communities, construing their identity from what they are and what they refuse to be. For instance, the cognitive-behavioral approach rejects the notion of the unconscious. In contrast, psychoanalysis denies the idea of a behavioral change that is not part of unconscious dynamic processes at work.

And yet, we can't leave it there as two separate communities with well-defined borders and a stable identity. The encounter must generate an affirmative answer: not just for the formation of self-identity and cultural ethos, but to bolster these. The act of welcoming a guest is also an opportunity to revisit one's own house. It situates the host within his own home and confirms its boundaries – precisely due to the questioning introduced by the guest's appearance. Here, the opposing schools have an opportunity to boost and endorse their views due to hospitality itself. An intelligent discourse between the host and the guest brings up questions and generates answers that reinforce the hosting tendency's perspectives and practices.

Let us imagine a cognitive-behavioral lecturer, an expert on anxiety disorders. A psychoanalytic institute invites her to give a talk. Even though some of the members have their doubts, they decide to attend. After all, they were the ones who invited the guest. And one owes a guest what the custom is under the rules of hospitality. The lecturer presents the techniques in which research has proven to be most effective in treating the disorder. The encounter aims not to cause psychoanalysts to abandon the worldviews they believe in but rather to better understand their approach, albeit from a different perspective. For instance, one might perceive interpretation as exposure to painful emotions or problematic relations and improvement in terms of practice and adjustment. Members of the psychoanalytic institute gain further confirmation of how their treatment can help patients in ways they did not foresee. Similarly, when members of the cognitive-behavioral approach invite a psychodynamic speaker to lecture on the subject of anxiety, and she proceeds to underline unconscious conflict, internalized object relations, and the defence mechanisms at work, they have a chance to understand their own work on patterns of thinking or behavior, as producing a change in these additional intrapsychic layers.

Moreover, for Derrida, the question of the other opens the possibility to expand the home. The encounter following an act of hospitality carries the potential gain of creative development for the hosting orientation. Under certain conditions, which we will discuss later, the invited school may leave behind ideas and practices that are productive and can inspire new ideas within the host's existing frame. The psychodynamic lecturer who speaks to an audience of cognitive-behavioral practitioners and trainees may present interpretations for a patient who is always late to his session while explaining transference processes and their contribution to interpretive techniques. The cognitive-behavioral therapists, having experienced similar problems with some of their patients, may gain ideas about these late arrivals' meaning and deploy this interpretive technique within their current theoretical frame. That is, they try to understand patterns of changes in terms of ways of thinking and behavior.

The same applies to the psychodynamically oriented audience who attend the lecture by the cognitive-behaviorist on, for example, gradual exposure to anxiety. The psychotherapists can use this technique in their psychodynamic work while taking a profound account of the patient's needs and object relations. Such encounters enable new ideas about therapy and are likely to expand existing knowledge on each hosting tendency. The approach that has been invited in, it is worth remembering, also stands to gain. As members of the audience belonging to the other school share their thoughts with the lecturer, she realizes that her technique is open to various interpretations and applications. In this way, the encounter enriches her too.

Hence, hospitality offers an occasion for self-examination no less than an acquaintance with the other. It might help confirm the hosting school in its answers and its cultural ethos while equally contributing to keeping its boundaries alive. Returning to the audience of psychoanalysts attending a lecture given by a cognitive-behavioral-oriented speaker on anxiety: institute members have an opportunity to check themselves in terms of the introduced ideas. Some of them will end up feeling confirmed in their beliefs, finding they now understand something new about themselves. Others might recollect a time when they had to work with a disorder of this type and discover they have gained a unique insight about it – for instance, the method they had believed to be working well had been successful for different reasons than they thought. Others may decide to refer patients suffering from this disorder to short-term treatment with the newly presented method or incorporate an idea they found useful in their therapy. Yet others may be prompted to reflect on how limited the use of a psychoanalytic approach is for this type of problem, encouraging them to find new ways to understand this lacuna. All this, however, can only happen on one condition: The audience must not feel threatened; they must not think that their professional identity is being questioned, interfering with the very foundations of their home.

What? – The Conditions for Hospitality

Considering the risks of hospitality, we must ask: What conditions allow such hospitality? As mentioned, pure hospitality, as it is defined under the ethical law, can be damaging:

> For unconditional hospitality to take place you have to accept the risk of the other coming and destroying the place, initiating a revolution, stealing everything, or killing everyone. That is the risk of pure hospitality and pure gift, because a pure gift might be terrible too (Derrida, 1999, p. 71).

Hospitality between the competing schools in psychotherapy is therefore threatened by impending dangers such as internal revolution, foreign overtake, assimilation, conversion, and even destruction of the cultural ethos. The guest who the competing school is hosting is under a similar threat. Ethical hospitality alone, completely unconditional, hence, is not possible and amounts to absolute madness. Hospitality always remains alive to traces of potential war and cannot but be conditional. One must, in other words, approach the intellectual and theoretical other and lend an ear to different voices; at the same time, one should act responsibly by checking out which alien elements may be admitted to the home's cultural narratives and by articulating conditions and constraints (Still, 2010). It is the school that undertakes the hosting, the "master of the house," that is the sovereign setting the rules of this meeting: the invitation's timing, what the guest may bring along, and what it might carry in – which ideas and practices, and on which specific topics it is welcome to discuss. When the psychoanalytic institute, for instance, invites a guest lecture from a cognitive-behavioral therapist, the invitation is to a specific speaker, who is welcome to join at a particular time and place, and discuss an agreed topic.

Therefore, to begin with, an invitation to receive a guest is needed, which, subsequently, requires the invitee's positive response to the host (Derrida, 2000). This mutual agreement – to host and be hosted –is needed if hospitality and an encounter occur. It is most likely that when such an invitation is not accepted, and the guest independently decides on the terms of the encounter, he or she will probably be perceived as an intruder.

Indeed, many therapists within the schools thought that "intruders" from different schools should stay away from their conceptual territory. For example, throughout the history of psychoanalysis, there have been voices calling to keep the discipline "pure" (Milton, 2001), untainted by foreign elements that will introduce assimilation and erode its particular identity. Such existential fear of invasion, assimilation, and destruction seems to have marked all the moments in psychoanalysis history even when thinkers from its midst proposed change (e.g., the controversies between Melanie Klein and Anna Freud, and others, as described in Govrin, 2015). On the other side, there have been similar calls to keep out psychoanalysis from training, research, and the public domain (Nouvel Observateur, 22 October 2019). An American colleague told me (Govrin, A., personal communication) about a written sign in a public mental health clinic staff room, reading: "Psychodynamic and any other techniques that are not evidence-based are not allowed here." Hence, the mutual lack of recognition between the two schools is not only due to their disagreement about different world views on therapy and its evaluation, or competition over public resources, and recognition and prestige, as mentioned before. We emphasize here that this is also the result of an existential fear of losing their respective identity and distinctiveness.

The following condition to hospitality answers this puzzle: hospitality does not involve similarity, fusion, or unification. It looks at the other, and the foreign – and this otherness is a necessary condition. For a relationship of hospitality with the other, we must assume distance and separateness between the two camps:

> The other is infinitely other because we never have any access to the other as such. That is why he/she is the other. This separation, this dissociation is not only a limit, but it is also the condition of the relation to the other, a nonrelation as relation (Derrida, 1999, p. 71).

This is an important point. If therapists from both schools want hospitality to be successful, they must acknowledge and cultivate their distinct and separate character. This way, the techniques of one approach and ideas will not be considered a part of the hosting approach, even when they are made intelligible and deployed in her language. In this manner, the fear of assimilation, conversion, unification, or annihilation is addressed.

How? – The Implementation of Hospitality

Finally, there are questions regarding the possibilities of implementing hospitality between the two competing schools. The first of these is about the kind of currently available options and what additional, practical opportunities this type of encounter holds.

Hospitality may take many forms, and it is always the product of a negotiation between the law of ethics and the political laws that condition it. For example, within the integration movement, it is practiced within the assimilative integration model: "… in which techniques or perspectives from other therapies are incorporated into a 'home' therapy" (Messer, 2019, p. 73). This type of integration requires a firm grounding in one psychotherapeutic system and openness to selectively include practices and views deriving from another system (Norcross & Alexander, 2019). The psychodynamic assimilation model (Stricker & Gold, 2019) and the cognitive-behavioral assimilative integration model (Castonguay, Newman & Holtforth, 2019), two of the most influential models of integration, for instance, are intellectually solidly reliant on and faithful to their respective, original theories. Adhering to their mother tongue and home ground enables them to direct their hospitality to specific components of the competing perspective. The latter is perceived as offering ways to expand the traditional model, though other elements are rejected and remain outside. In doing so, they maintain the tension between ethical and political laws and represent different hospitality expressions in psychotherapy.

For clinicians to further "open their doors" to the other rival school, it is essential that, from the outset, the encounter should not present itself as a dispute or an attempt to reduce differences. It should set itself up as a meeting between hosts who come to listen and talk with guests and engage in an honest debate allowing for both disagreement and openness. We would like to suggest that each time one of the schools takes the stage on study days or conferences, a competing school representative will be invited to offer their perspective. Hospitality can also be practiced in written form – in journals or in books – when the other side is asked to present its views on the issue in question. And it can enter professional training institutes through their curricula, which might invite from time to time to host professionals from the other school. As Messer and Winokur (1980) argue, psychotherapy students in all study programmes must be exposed to both orientations' theories and practices.

We believe, therefore, that hospitality can be exercised at any level we choose: in the discussion about our worldview and theory, about our practices, research, training, and writing as long as we keep the tension of the double law – between ethics and politics. On the one hand, the objective is to gain respect and familiarity with other ways of thinking and conducting therapy and allow for a degree of mutual influence between them. At the same time, the aim is to fortify each therapeutic approach on this basis.

Two Obstacles for Hospitality

So far, most of our argument was concerned with protecting the psychotherapist's professional identity ("home") while still maintaining an open approach to foreign practice. However, psychotherapists from both camps might tackle two other problems that might hinder the host and the guest's mutual influence. First, if the host and the guest perceive the differences between them as unbridgeable, it might be impossible to form an open-minded attitude. Indeed, CBT and psychoanalysis hold two opposing worldviews on essential questions: What is a human being's nature? What are the aims of psychotherapy? What is the place of affect, motivation, and cognition in psychopathology? The obstacle of unresolvable disagreements is different from the barrier of identity. Whereas hosting a stranger threatens the group's cohesion and identity, bringing two groups who hold opposing views might threaten each group's convictions and firm beliefs. This might lead to strong opposition and even contempt as a defence against doubt.

The American philosopher, logician, and scientist Charles Peirce wrote in the "Fixation of belief" (1877):

> Doubt is an uneasy and dissatisfied state from which we struggle to free our-selves and pass into the state of belief; while the latter is a calm and satisfactory state which we do not wish to avoid, or to change to a belief in anything else. On the contrary, we cling tenaciously, not merely to believing, but to believing just what we do believe (p. 3).

Psychotherapists who hold firm convictions on subjects like the aim of psycho-therapy might feel that other contrasting views violently invalidate their lived experience or distort the facts of events they have witnessed during their clinical experience. These psychotherapists do not share Peirce's commitment to fallibi-lism, which "requires a man to be at all times ready to dump his whole cart-load of beliefs, the moment experience is against them" (CP 1.55, 1896, in: Peirce, 1931). At first glance, the use of the notion of hospitality to enhance mutual influence can accommodate only those who believe that inquiry should continue indefinitely and that healthy doubt is part of scientific exploration. However, we believe that guests' and hosts' role is likely to enhance tolerance to differences and disagreements even among the most zealous psychotherapists. As guests, they will be motivated to impact their hosts by presenting what they perceive as profoundly new ways of thinking about effective interventions and successful psychotherapeutic outcomes. As hosts, they might feel a background of safety in their home's comfort zones, which is more likely to enable them to avoid their usual response of pushing aside in condensation the "foreign" ideas and instead show more interest and curiosity.

The second obstacle for the notion of hospitality is the problem of language. Many theoretical concepts have a history, or a subtle connotation, in a given theory that may be different or completely absent in another approach, so it might not be easy for the host and guest to understand their ideas in their original meaning. Practitioners of both schools can sometimes use different terms to describe quite similar phenomena (e.g., early maladaptive schemas and internalized object relations in Young, Klo-sko & Weishaar, 2003). The same words can also be used to describe different and only partially overlapping phenomena (e.g., the discussion on the concept of self and how theorists use it in different ways in Mascolo & Maheshwari, 2019).

Achieving perfect translation is impossible for another reason. Hospitality always takes place in language and is conditioned on agreement formulated in the host's language, who will attempt to understand something about the other in their language. This means that the host imposes herself on the hosted other. When one school hosts the other, it conducts the conversation in its familiar language. It understands the other school's ideas and concepts through this language. We believe that the hosted school should accept its role as a guest and come to terms with this distortion. Like poets who permit translation of their poems into another language knowing that meanings will be lost in translation, psychotherapists must accept that their ideas and concepts will lose some of their original meaning when translated into the other's language.

So, when the psychodynamic approach acts as host, the speaker on CBT therapy talking about anxiety disorder will most likely be understood in terms of unconscious conflict and internalized object relations, and how they affect the emotional experience, interpersonal relations, and functioning. Similarly, a speaker who is an expert on anxiety from a psychodynamic perspective will agree to be understood by a CBT audience in CBT terms and accept that her ideas will be translated into CBT theories and techniques.

In fact, translation between two different approaches is both likely and unlikely, both humble and violent. Humble because the host is sincere in his or her efforts to understand the other approach's perspective in a way that would be loyal to the guest. Violent because once the host is engaged in absorbing the new material, he cannot help but distort it and reduce it to the language he or she is familiar with. But the important point is that this is also an opportunity for both the host and the guest: hospitality creates multiple associations of meaning and different types of interpretations in translation. Various interpretations can make room for discovering and broadening the breadth of the host's theory. In doing so, each of these schools will, on the one hand, preserve their distinct identities, intelligently boosting their cultural ethos, and, on the other, open their doors to vital and enriching development.

Note

1 In Israel, as in other countries, the establishment of each school remains extremely orthodox (Shahar, 2011b), but university departments of clinical psychology are diverse. In the UK, many psychological therapy departments include a range of psychotherapeutic approaches which do not necessarily either have a primary orientation or explicitly integrative perspective. These forms are less controversial because the practitioners do not feel a strong sense of loyalty to one approach. However, the model we present here is recommended for those who strongly resist change outside their own school, the most loyal supporters of each school.

References

Anchin, J.C. (2008) Contextualizing discourse on a philosophy of science for psychotherapy integration. *Journal of Psychotherapy Integration* 18(1): 1–24.

Arkowitz, H. & Messer, S.B. (eds) (1984) *Psychoanalytic Therapy and Behavior Therapy: Is Integration Possible?*. New York: Plenum.

Beck, A.T. (1976) *Cognitive Therapy and the Emotional Disorders*. New York: International Universities Press.

Blagys, M.D. & Hilsenroth, M.J. (2000) Distinctive features of short-term psychodynamic interpersonal psychotherapy: A review of the comparative psychotherapy process literature. *Clinical Psychology: Science and Practice* 7: 167–88.

Blagys, M.D. & Hilsenroth, M.J. (2002) Distinctive activities of cognitive-behavioral therapy. A review of the comparative psychotherapy process literature. *Clinical Psychology Review* 22: 671–706.

Butler, A.C., Chapman, J.E.F., Evan, M. & Beck, A. (2006) The empirical status of cognitive-behavioral therapy: A review of meta-analyses. *Clinical Psychology Review* 26 (1): 17–31.

Cambridge Dictionary, online edition, s.v. 'hospitality'. Available at: https://dictionary.cambridge.org/dictionary/english/hospitality (accessed 21 July 2020).

Castonguay, L.G., Newman, M.G. & Holtforth, M.G. (2019) Cognitive-behavioral assimilative integration. In: Norcross, J. C. & Goldfried, M. R. (eds), *Handbook of Psychotherapy Integration*, pp. 228–51. New York: Oxford University Press.

Cook, M.J., Biyanova, T., Elhai, J., Schnurr, P.P. & Coyne, J.C. (2010) What do psychotherapists really do in practice? An internet study of over 2,000 practitioners. *Psychotherapy: Theory, Research, Practice, Training* 47(2): 260–7.

Crits-Christoph, P., Wilson, G.T. & Hollon, S.D. (2005) Empirically supported psychotherapies: Comment on Westen, Novotny, and Thompson-Brenner (2004). *Psychological Bulletin 131*(3): 412–17.

Derrida, J. (1991) 'Eating well', or the calculation of the subject: An interview with Jacques Derrida. In: Cadava, E., Connor, P. & Nancy, J.- L. (eds), *Who Comes After the Subject?*. New York and London: Routledge.

Derrida, J. (1997a) *Adieu a Emmanuel Levinas* (trans. Brault, P- A. & Naas, M.). Redwood City: Stanford University Press, 1999.

Derrida, J. (1997b) *Of Hospitality* (trans. Bowlby, R.). Redwood City: Stanford University Press, 2000.

Derrida, J. (1999) Hospitality, justice and responsibility: A dialogue with Jacques Derrida. In: Kearney, R. & Dooley, M. (eds), *Questioning Ethics: Contemporary Debates in Philosophy*, pp. 65–83. London: Routledge.

Derrida, J. (2000) Hospitality. *Angeloki* 5(3): 3–18.

Derrida, J. (2001) On cosmopolitanism. In: *On Cosmopolitanism and Forgiveness* (trans. Dooley, M. & Hughes, M.), pp. 16–17. London and New York: Routledge.

Derrida, J. (2004) *Abraham's Melancholy: Interview with Jacques Derrida*. Michal Ben-Naftali. Tel Aviv: Resling, 2016.

Derrida, J. (2005) The principle of hospitality. In: *Paper Machine* (trans. Bowlby, R.), pp. 66–9. Redwood City: Stanford University Press.

Downing, J.N. (2004) Psychotherapy practice in a pluralistic world: Philosophical and moral dilemmas. *Journal of Psychotherapy Integration* 14(2): 123–48.

Edelstein, M.R., Kujoth, R.K. & Ramsay Steele, D. (2013) *Therapy Breakthrough: Why Some Psychotherapies Work Better Than Others*. Chicago: Open Court Publishing.

Ellis, A. (1962) *Reason and Emotion in Psychotherapy*. New York, NY: Lyle Stuart.

Freud, S. (1913) *The Interpretations of Dreams*. New York: Macmillan.

Freud, S. (1919) Ways of the psychoanalytical therapy. In: Berman, E. & Rolnik, E. J. (eds), *Psychoanalytic Treatment* (trans. Rolnik, E.J.), pp. 129–35.Tel-Aviv: Am-Oved, 2003.

Gardner, J.R. (2017) Divergence and convergence: An examination of cognitive–behavioral and dynamic therapies, theoretical and clinical perspectives. *Journal of Psychotherapy Integration* 27(3): 395–406.

Glover, E. (1931) The therapeutic effect of inexact interpretation: A contribution to the theory of suggestion. *International Journal of Psychoanalysis* 12: 397–411.

Goldfried, M.R., Pachankis, J.E. & Goodwin, B.J. (2019) A history of psychotherapy integration. In: Norcross, J. C. & Goldfried, M. R. (eds), *Handbook of Psychotherapy Integration*, pp. 28–63.New York: Oxford University Press.

Govrin, A. (2015) *Conservative and Radical Perspectives on Psychoanalytic Knowledge: The Fascinated and the Disenchanted*. London: Routledge.

Hofmann, S.G. & Smits, J.A. (2017) The evolution of cognitive behavioral therapy for anxiety and depression. *Psychiatric Clinics of North America* 40(4): 11–12.

Jones, E.E. & Pulos, S.M. (1993) Comparing the process in psychodynamic and cognitive behavioral therapies. *Journal of Consulting and Clinical Psychology* 61: 306–16.

Kafka, F. (2009) *The Castle* (trans. Bell, A., introduction and notes by Robertson, R.), p. 15. Oxford: Oxford University Press.

Kubacki, S.R. & Chase, M. (1998) Comparing values and methods in psychodynamic and cognitive-behavioral therapy: Commonalities and differences. *Journal of Psychotherapy Integration* 8(1): 1–25.

Kubie, L.S. (1934) Relation of the conditioned reflex to psychoanalytic technic. *Archives of Neurology and Psychiatry* 32: 1137–42.

Laska, K.M., Gurman, A.S. & Wampold, B.E. (2014) Expanding the lens of evidence-based practice in psychotherapy: A common factors perspective. *Psychotherapy* 51(4): 467–81.

Leichsenring, F., Leweke, F., Klein, S. & Steinert, C. (2015) Empirical status of psychodynamic psychotherapy – an update: Bambi's alive and kicking. *Psychotherapy and Psychosomatics* 84(3): 129–48.

Leuzinger-Bohleber, M., Stuhr, U., Rüger, B. & Beutel, M.(2003) How to study the 'quality of psychoanalytic treatments' and their long-term effects on patients' well-being: A representative, multi-perspective follow-up study. *International Journal of Psychoanalysis* 84 (2): 263–90.

Levinas, E. (1961) *Totality and Infinity: An Essay on Exteriority* (trans. Lingis, A.). Pittsburgh: Duquesne University Press, 1969.

Levinas, E. (1974) *Otherwise than Being or Beyond Essence* (trans. Lingis, A.). Dordrecht: Kluwer Academic Publishers, 1978.

Lewis, E.C. (1970) *The Psychology of Counseling*. Oxford: Holt, Rinehart & Winston.

Mahoney, M.J. (2005) Suffering, philosophy, and psychotherapy. *Journal of Psychotherapy Integration* 15(3): 337–51.

Marom, S. (2010) Is there a place for psychoanalysis in Israel today? *MEDICINE Israeli journal of Psychiatry* 14: 10–13.

Mascolo, M.F. & Maheshwari, S. (2019) Images of self in psychological thought. *Psychological Studies* 64: 249–57.

Messer, S.B. (1986) Behavioral and psychoanalytic perspectives at therapeutic choice points. *American Psychologist* 41: 1261–72.

Messer, S.B. (2019) My journey through psychotherapy integration by twists and turns. *Journal of Psychotherapy Integration* 29(2): 73–83.

Messer, S.B. & Winokur, M. (1980) Some limits to the integration of psychoanalytic and behavior therapy. *American Psychologist* 35: 818–27.

Milton, J. (2001) Psychoanalysis and cognitive behavior therapy – rival paradigms or common ground? *International Journal of Psychoanalysis* 82: 431–46.

Norcross, J.C. & Alexander, E.F. (2019) A primer on psychotherapy integration. In: Norcross, J. C. & Goldfried, M. R. (eds), *Handbook of Psychotherapy Integration*, pp. 3–27. New York: Oxford University Press.

Peirce, C.S. (1877) The fixation of belief. *Popular Science Monthly* 12(November): 1–15.

Peirce, C.S. (1931) *Collected Papers*, Vol. 1–6 (eds Hartshorne and Weiss), pp. 7–8. Cambridge: Harvard University Press, 1935.

Rosner, R.I. (2002) Aaron T. Beck's dream theory in context: An introduction to his 1971 article on cognitive patterns in dreams and daydreams. *Journal of Cognitive Psychotherapy* 16(1): 7–22.

Rosner, R.I. (2012) Aaron T. Beck's drawings and the psychoanalytic origin story of cognitive therapy. *History of Psychology* 15(1): 1–18.

Safran, J.D. & Messer, S.B. (1997) Psychotherapy integration: A postmodern critique. *Clinical Psychology: Science & Practice* 4: 140–52.

Schoenfeld, E. (2007). Introduction. In: Derrida, J. (ed.), *Of Hospitality*, pp. 7–16. Tel Aviv: Resling.

Shahar, G. (2011a) Introduction. In: N. Mor, J. Meijers, S. Marom and E. Gilboa-Schechtman (Eds.). *Cognitive Behavioral Therapy for Adults: Therapeutic Principals*. Tel-Aviv: Probook.

Shahar, G. (2011b) Israeli clinical psychology – where to? *Conversations – Israeli Journal of Psychotherapy* 26(1): 1–7.

Shedler, J. (2010) The efficacy of psychodynamic psychotherapy. *American Psychologist* 65 (2): 98–109.

Shedler J. (2015) Where is the evidence for 'evidence based' psychotherapy? The *Journal for Psychological Therapies in Primary Care* 4: 47–59.

Skinner, B.F. (1953) *Science and Human Behavior*. New York: Macmillan.

Steinert, C., Munder, T., Rabung, S., Hoyer, J. & Leichsenring, F. (2017) Psychodynamic therapy: As efficacious as other empirically supported treatments? A meta-analysis testing equivalence of outcomes. *The American Journal of Psychiatry* 174(10): 943–53.

Still, J. (2010) *Derrida and Hospitality Theory and Practice*. Edinburgh: Edinburgh University Press.

Stricker, G. (2010) A second look at psychotherapy integration. Journal of Psychotherapy Integration 20(4): 397–405.

Stricker, G. & Gold, J.R. (2019) Assimilative psychodynamic psychotherapy. In: Norcross, J. C. & Goldfried, M. R. (eds), *Handbook of Psychotherapy Integration*, pp. 207–27. New York: Oxford University Press.

Wachtel, P.L. (2010) Psychotherapy integration and integrative psychotherapy: Process or product? *Journal of Psychotherapy Integration* 20(4): 406–16.

Wachtel, P.L. (2018) Pathways to progress for integrative psychotherapy: Perspectives on practice and research. *Journal of Psychotherapy Integration* 28(2): 202–12.

Walter, B. (1946) *Theme and Variations: An Autobiography*. New York: A.A. Knopf.

Wampold, B.E. & Ulvenes, P.G. (2019) Integration of common factors and specific ingredients. In: Norcross, J. C. & Goldfried, M. R. (eds), *Handbook of Psychotherapy Integration*. New York, Oxford University Press. p. 69–87.

Westen, D., Novotny, C.M. & Thompson-Brenner, H. (2004) The empirical status of empirically supported psychotherapies: Assumptions, findings, and reporting in controlled clinical trials. *Psychological Bulletin* 130(4): 631–63.

Wolpe, J. (1969) *The Practice of Behavior Therapy*. Oxford: Pergamon Press.

Young, J.E., Klosko, J.S. & Weishaar, M.E. (2003) *Schema Therapy: A Practitioner's Guide*. New York: The Guilford Press.

Zilcha-Mano, S. & Errázuriz, P. (2015) One size does not fit all: Examining heterogeneity and identifying moderators of the alliance–outcome association. *Journal of Counseling Psychology* 62(4): 579–91.

Ziv-Beiman, S. & Shahar, G. (2014) What is integrative psychotherapy? *Conversations Israeli Journal of Psychotherapy* 28(2): 156–63.

Chapter 3

Dialectical Integration – The Case of Psychoanalysis and Cognitive-Behavioral Therapy

Yael Peri Herzovich and Aner Govrin

Based on Hegel's dialectics, we argue in this chapter that different psychotherapies considered monolithic such as cognitive-behavioral therapy (CBT) and psychoanalysis, even though they hold radically different views on human suffering and therapy's aims, profoundly influence each other. We call this mutual influence dialectical integration (DI). DI is the result of unconscious processes that are activated by antagonism and negation for self-constitution. In a dialectically formative process, the self-constitution of CBT and psychoanalysis each is achieved by means of the negation of part of itself, which undergoes alienation in the other, thereby superficially taking the form of a rejection of the other approach. But whenever theoretical or practical lacunae occur in the unfolding of these disciplines, they negate this primary negation and re-internalize the alienated self-component. This part does not return in its original – and negated – form, but through a sublation introducing theoretical and practical development. This is illustrated here by Hartmann's ego psychology, Beck's cognitive theory, Young's schema therapy, and Bateman and Fonagy's mentalization-based therapy (MBT). We show how these developments incorporate elements of otherness, which are not simply extraneous to the tradition but also part of it. We conclude by showing how DI gives rise to recognition and containment of otherness in both schools.

Integration in Psychotherapy as a Combination of Approaches

The effort toward integration in psychotherapy seeks to combine key approaches on the assumption that no one type of therapy can offer a solution to all challenges. There currently exist a variety of integrative psychotherapies, which differ in terms of the approaches they combine and how they link theory and practice. The four most popular routes are technical eclecticism, theoretical integration, common factors, and assimilative integration. All four routes are characterized by a general desire to increase therapeutic efficacy, efficiency, and applicability by looking beyond the confines of single theories and the restricted techniques traditionally associated with those theories. They follow from a general perspective that includes acceptance of the other, setting aside rigid ideological differences for

DOI: 10.4324/9781003608103-4

the sake of flexibility and a fundamental commitment to the best possible solutions for the patient. The outcome is a pluralistic approach that resists any therapeutic community or position that lays claim on one truth, whether in the theoretical or practical context (Norcross & Alexander, 2019).

Supporters of integrative approaches are perceived as open-minded, permeable, flexible, pluralistic, and keen on cooperation and fusion, while those who adhere to one approach are considered purists, monolithic, and hermetic. This chapter shows how integration, permeability, and influence also occur within non-pluralistic approaches – but here, they unfold through dialectical processes that guide self-constitution. To illustrate, we will examine a long-standing intense antagonism in the field of psychotherapy: the relations between psychoanalysis and CBT.

Since both schools emerged in the field, they have undergone many theoretical evolutions. For example, there have been many developments within CBT since the behavioral basis for the approach, like cognitive development, and theories associated with the "third wave," such as act and schema therapy. However, common core principles among these approaches emphasize maladaptive thought processes and behaviors (Hayes, 2004).

Psychoanalysis also developed since Freud's time to ego psychology, object relation theory, self-psychology, relationality, and intersubjectivity psychology (Boswell et al., 2010). There is often a bitter debate within psychoanalysis about what psychoanalysis is (Blass, 2010a). It is customary to refer to the nucleus of the identity of psychoanalysis as lies in the "understanding" of unconscious dynamics (Migone, 2011).

The assumption that psychoanalysis is a rival to CBT implies the presumption that psychoanalysis is indeed therapy. This question of psychoanalysis as a therapy occupies psychoanalysts and leads to many disagreements (Blass, 2010b). Migone(2011) argues that psychoanalysis should be defined as a theory, not a technique, and that different techniques are applications of that theory. So, in considering the relationship between analysis and therapy, one must wonder about the aims that guide the analyst or therapist and how they shape the method and its analytic or nonanalytic character. Migone argues that if different techniques are applications of a defined theory, then the difference between psychoanalysis and psychoanalytic psychotherapy melts away: "in order to be analysts, with a given patient, we need to be psychotherapists" (p. 1316).

The rivalry between these two major forces seems to involve two clashing extremes. First, they are committed to different worldviews and ways of understanding the human psyche, suffering, therapy definitions, practices, and envisioned processes (Kubacki & Chase, 1998). Second, although both approaches have evolved and have absorbed different therapeutic tendencies and methods – which among themselves often fail to reach an agreement, loyalties to one of the traditions usually tend to position themselves extremely critically and even censoriously in the face of the rival approach (for criticism of CBT, see, for instance, Miltone, 2001; and for criticism of psychoanalysis, see Edelstein, Kujoth & Ramsey Steele, 2013).

In these circumstances, it is difficult to attain the kind of open-mindedness and communication between the approaches that would enable them to reflect on themselves and learn from each other, let alone to consciously and intentionally adopt elements from each other. It is important to say that we are aware of the intensive successful attempts to integrate the two theories. But, besides these conscious and directed attempts, we point to another hidden influence occurring between the two that we believe shaped the two schools.

The DI process that we propose in this chapter, unlike in declared integrative approaches, is not a conscious process. Here the foreign element is not taken on board with an intentionally integrative motivation. DI is the result of unconscious processes that are activated by antagonism and negation for self-constitution.

The critical point is that this unconscious process of receiving foreign elements includes foreign components that are also self-components. We argue here that each approach already contains the other's otherness, which is nothing but its own otherness. When Freud (1919a) writes about the uncanny (the recurrence of something long forgotten and repressed), he claims that the uncanny is nothing new or alien but something familiar and long established in the mind that has become alienated from it only through the process of repression. Kristeva (1991) refers to the Freudian definition of the uncanny and argues that what we consider foreign – which manifests as hatred of the other – includes a hidden aspect of our identity. The difficulty we have in accepting the other, she believes, is the outcome of our inability to acknowledge our subjective otherness. The hatred of the stranger manifests the unconscious projection and rejection of threatening materials that were removed from ourselves. The result is that what we experience as a threatening other is not only his or her foreignness but the foreignness of ourselves.

To demonstrate how the external element of otherness preexists in each of the two approaches in the form of an internal, inherent part that is neither intentional nor conscious, we introduce an epistemological and ontological foundation for encountering the other through Hegelian dialectics. We claim that these two psychotherapeutic methods entertain dialectical relations that are more complicated than we would expect, in which each of their courses of development as a separate monolithic body depends on the other. This implies that integration also occurs in a monolithic domain and that ostensibly monolithic approaches undergo the influence of different approaches. The vital formation and existence of each of them depend dynamically on that of the other.

Two crucial developments in the field are discussed here in order to follow this dialectic: Hartmann's ego psychology in the psychoanalytic approach and the development of Beck's cognitive theory in the cognitive-behavioral approach. Then, we will briefly demonstrate such a dialectical development in two recent developments: schema therapy in CBT and MBT in psychoanalysis. Earlier, we defined the common core principles in each school. Based on the principles mentioned earlier, these representative models were selected.

Below we introduce Hegel's dialectics to provide a groundwork, both ontological and epistemological, for thinking about the development of these psychotherapeutic approaches as a scientific subject and body of knowledge with an inner development that contains unconscious otherness and foreignness. This chapter cannot do justice to Hegel's complex and comprehensive dialectics. Instead, we shall limit ourselves to some of its key concepts.

Hegel's Method

Hegel's dialectics addresses the question of the growth of scientific knowledge (Cohen & Wartofsky, 1984). Thagard (1982) argues that one can form an apparent understanding of how Hegel's dialectics construes the growth of scientific knowledge from the dialectics of the stages of consciousness, as they appear in *The Phenomenology of Spirit* (Hegel, 2018), in which he foregrounds the human subject's development of knowledge.

We first describe the dialectical process of the formation of the subject. Then we describe the development of a subject-like system that is obtained for the process of knowledge consolidation.

Dialectics as Subject Formation

Dialectics is introduced principally in *The Phenomenology of Spirit*. It is described as a process or even journey through which self-consciousness and self-knowledge evolve using mutual recognition of or with the other, that is, with the mediation of the other. According to Hegel, self-consciousness exists for [another] consciousness. That is, self-consciousness is defined by its being recognized as self-conscious by another self-consciousness. This means that being a free agent consists of being recognized as one. However, at the same time, Hegel values self-determination, which suggests fundamental independence from others (Burke, 2005).

Consciousness, for Hegel, is not initially of the self but of something other, an object. Consciousness relates to this object as what is not itself, and this essential duality defines it. As a result of recognizing another object, consciousness comes to know itself (Hegel calls this state of consciousness "in itself"). Self-consciousness, in contrast, is consciousness whose object is itself, and it presents its contents to itself as an object. Here, in other words, the subject is its own object, a subject that simultaneously determines itself as a conscious object of this determination (this state of consciousness Hegel calls "for itself"; Klein, 1978).

We can describe the process through which consciousness evolves into self-consciousness: the dialectical point of departure is that self-consciousness, in order to realize itself as self-consciousness, requires another self-consciousness to restore it to itself. In this process, in order to consolidate reflexivity, consciousness must move outside itself to acquire objective status through the other's recognition. This outward movement of self-consciousness is enabled by its being an infinite negation of what it is. The initial outcome of this negation is the bifurcation of consciousness within its own boundaries. As a result of this splitting, consciousness no longer experiences itself as whole or monolithic and becomes other to itself. It maintains its identity by casting its alterity away from and out of itself.

This otherness is externalized in another self-consciousness. Self-consciousness becomes self-alienated in putting its own otherness into another being. In so doing, it cancels the other self-consciousness: this act does not recognize the other self-consciousness as an autonomous entity. Instead, it sees itself in this other self-consciousness. It is not, at this point, aware that the otherness it observes is nothing but itself. The experience, instead, is of a foreign other. Self-consciousness expects that the other passively reflects it – self-consciousness – back to itself. The other self-consciousness, however, is also seeking itself in the – first – self-consciousness. Consciousness, to "discover" itself "for itself," returns to itself by cancelling its alienated self in the other. Removing itself from the other also restores the other to itself (Kenan, 2019).

The dialectic process then includes three moves or stages: (1) initial identity; (2) negation of the initial identity, resulting in difference; and (3) negation of the negation, resulting in renewed identity that leads to a new and more complex identity. In every dialectical development, the subject matter's primary form is negated and cancelled, while its original meaning is preserved at a structurally and discursively higher level, a component in a novel situation – and this is what is called sublation – from the German Aufhebung which suggests negation, conservation, and elevation or progress (Yovel, 2005). Each stage sublates the previous one and takes its place in the process of constantly rising levels.

The result is that consciousness evolves into self-consciousness with a dialectical identity whose essence is the unity of identity and difference. This is, in other words, a consciousness with a unifying structure that turns the plurality of its expressions into a continuous and ongoing narrative mediated through otherness. In this process, self-consciousness emerges as a condition in which it is in and for itself. "In and for itself" refers to the mode of being of a system that has realized its essence by externalizing itself in its opposing other and then returning to itself. This affords it a dimension of being ("in itself") and a dimension of reflection ("for itself") – dimensions which fulfil themselves within this self-consciousness and are responsible for its dialectical identity.

Dialectics as the Development of Knowledge

As mentioned, Hegel's dialectics, over and beyond describing the development of the human subject, also articulates the process of epistemological development of knowledge as a system resembling the human subject. For Hegel, absolute being (or knowledge), too, taking the shape of the subject, rather than being what it is right from the outset, proceeds toward itself through its opposites: multiplicity and otherness, using negation. Moreover, like in the case of the subject, negation does not end at the point of departure but brings about a new state of affairs (state of consciousness). These negations do not erase earlier stages as the latter are inscribed in the very texture of the next stage, this renders what is called "sublation" (Yovel, 2005).

Sublation as a movement of dialectical development has three moments: the negation or cancellation of a given form, conservation of fundamental content, and elevation of this content to a more appropriate level of expression. In the process of sublation, certain elements are rejected to preserve and include essential elements. While preserving and maintaining, however, sublation also criticizes and sets itself free from earlier forms of thinking. Sublation always involves qualitative renewal as a result of which the subject is raised to a higher ontological level (Yovel, 1975). At any developmental point, the collapse of one position causes the process to advance toward a new position that serves as a specific answer, however temporary, to a specific lacuna that revealed itself at the earlier stage and caused its collapse.

The point of the dialectical process is to achieve the stage where contradictions no longer arise; this ultimate, self-sufficient stage is called absolute knowledge. Hegel assumed that knowledge converged to form a complete and full description of reality, which is realized in the "absolute." The absolute, for him, is an individual totality that knows itself by being restored to itself following its alienation in the other. In this return, it realizes its objective of seamless self-consciousness of the kind that knows itself in its otherness, but rather than from alienation, it is now a result of identification with this otherness of the self as the "unity of identity and difference."

Various criticisms have been made of Hegel's model, starting with difficulty reading Hegel's complicated writings, the circularity of his model, and the universal generalization he seeks to apply (Knowles, 1985). However, it should be mentioned that Hegel emerged from German idealism, which aims for total and absolute forms of explanation. In comparison, such complete and absolute forms are no longer acceptable in our postmodern era. Our interest in Hegel's ontology and epistemology focuses on the development of knowledge that takes the form of self-consciousness qua process and not with a wish to reach the end of that process.

We may ask, how does Hegel advance our cause? Mills (2012) claims that despite the criticism, Hegel's philosophy is particularly significant for the future of psychoanalysis. In our case, we will emphasize in his argument the significance to the field of psychotherapy. Hegel's great insight that reality – including every intellectual discipline – deals with process, evolution, and change out of mutual recognition leads to a new understanding of the historical development of essential tendencies in psychotherapy, as integrative in essence. That may lead to a new consideration between disciplines and bridge the gap between rival psychotherapeutic schools.

Below we employ Hegel's method to discuss how each school has affected the other's development resulting in a different view of integration: DI.

The Dialectical Development of Psychotherapies

The present DI between approaches in psychotherapy seeks to follow internal development in each of the approaches. According to Yovel (2005), the right philosophy illuminates the rational structure of the object itself from the inside and could not simply or schematically be applied to the material under consideration from the outside.

Coming at this dialectically, we will argue that the psychotherapeutic approaches, being subject-like epistemological structures, are evolving organic systems that sustain themselves using negation. In this way, they establish their cultural-professional identity and the knowledge they carry. Through a process of DI, the self-formation of each psychotherapeutic approach comes about by negating or rejecting part of itself which then is alienated in the other. This manifests, superficially, as a rejection of the other approach. For instance, the cognitive-behavioral approach rejects the notion of the unconscious. In contrast, psychoanalysis denies the idea of a behavioral change that is not part of unconscious dynamic processes at work. This move creates an "us-them" distinction and emphasizes salient differences to sustain professional-cultural identity (Peri Herzovich & Govrin, 2021).

But when lacunae appear in each approach's development, they negate the abovementioned primary negation to bring back the element of the self that underwent alienation. However, this returned element does not maintain its original, early, and negated form: it undergoes a sublation that adds theoretical as well as practical complexity and development.

In the dialectic process, even when one position refutes the one preceding it, this does not merely contradict it but, using sublation, preserves a moment of its otherness, and elevates it to the next level. Offering a solution to a specific deficiency enriches and completes the very principle it criticizes.

This process leads to the complex and evolved reincorporation of elements which are simultaneously elements of the self and the other. The internal development of each of the approaches, therefore, depends on the other in the process of its own, separate formation.

Dialectical Integration – The Case of Psychoanalysis and CBT

We will now illustrate chronological dialectical development processes in psychotherapeutic approaches by considering two central ones in the field. One is psychoanalysis in the face of Hartmann's ego psychology. The other is CBT and its dynamic with Beck's cognitive theory. Then, we will briefly demonstrate such a dialectical development in two recent developments: schema therapy in CBT and MBT in psychoanalysis. We will see that integration is an essential developmental component in both approaches, calling this DI.

Hartmann's Ego Psychology

Freud's structural model featured a clash between unconscious and conscious mental functioning, where the id's impulses push against the ego's defenses (Freud, 1923). In this model, the ego represented one of the three fundamental agencies of the psyche, along with the id and superego. The ego sets itself up to arbitrate between the demands of the id, the superego, and the outside world. For Freud, the ego's primary functions are to represent reality and channel and control internal pressures of the drives in the face of reality, including the demands of social and moral convention, by setting up defenses (Mitchell & Black, 1995).

Freud gave center stage to the conflictual duality that dominates human existence: gratification of drives versus recognition of reality. Hartmann (1939, 1964), generally considered the founder of ego psychology, reduced his psychology to centering on the individual's development toward adaptation to an external, objective reality devoid of conflict. In doing so, Hartmann intended to transform Freudian psychoanalysis from a complex perspective full of contradiction to a coherent and systematic one (Govrin, 2004).

Freud considered ego functions in the context of psychic conflict, in which unconscious instinctual drives are gratified through a secondary process rather than through a primary process involving an encounter with reality, implying that the ego develops at a later stage. Like Freud, Hartmann based his theory on Darwin's theory of evolution. However, Hartmann emphasized how the human organism, like all other organisms, adjusted and adapted to its environment. Thus, he proposed "conflict-free ego functions," which are innate potential functions in place from the start of life and will naturally manifest themselves in the appropriate environment to help the individual to adapt. These capacities include social skills, language, and cognition.

Dialectically, this can be seen as an influence from behavior therapy based on learning theories that were prevalent at the time and which psychoanalysis rejected. Behaviorism was based on Pavlov (classic conditioning), Thorndike (operant conditioning), and Watson (learning theory). Major figures associated with this school of thought were Wolpe (1969) and Skinner (1953). In response to psychoanalysis, behavior therapy emerged as an approach committed to developing well-specified and rigorously tested applied techniques based on scientifically well-established basic principles. Behavior therapists criticized the psychoanalytic fancy that could be occasioned by the simplest of phobias or other clinical disorders. The alternative presented by behavior therapy was direct, humble, rational, and empirical. Abandoning an interest in hypothesized unconscious fears and desires, behavior therapists focused instead on direct symptom relief. Clinical targets generally involved "first-order" change, like focusing on "good social skills," not unconscious interests or conflicts (Hayes, 2004).

Tryon (1986) indicated the influence of CBT on ego psychology and noted their similarities in that the latter looks at emotions, thoughts, and behaviors that are not the direct outcome of the conflict between the id and the superego. It sees behavioral problems from the point of view of compromised thinking patterns that emerge from adapting to the environment. It is an approach that dedicates itself more to problem-solving than does classical psychoanalysis. Like the behavioral learning approach, Hartmann deals relatively little with unconscious parts of human experience. Instead, it aims at conscious learning principles in the individual's ongoing attempt to adapt to their environment.

And yet Hartmann kept saying throughout his writing that he was not changing (what he understood to be) the fundamental ideas of Freud's theory but rather expanding on them. Arguably he fully accepts the biological and evolutionary ideas in Freud's metapsychology, and he considers this the very core of psychoanalysis. In this model, however, the ego features as a primary adaptive development that is non-conflictual. He did not simply ignore conflicts but rather argued that defenses that initially emerge from conflict might, over time, become autonomous due to the development of adaptive ability. Hartmann (1939) wanted to adhere to the tradition and stay faithful to classical psychoanalysis. In his writings, he makes a point of referring to Freud's writings on thinking (p. 59). And along with this, he rejects nonanalytical theories which limit themselves to the role of behavior or cognition:

> The functions of intelligence appear, as a rule, in a different light in the course of psychoanalysis than in this attempt to isolate them ... we see intellectual achievements as both tools of conflict solving and of rationalizing and consider them in relation to the demands of the external world and the superego and, of course, in their interaction with other ego functions (p. 62).

It is illuminating to approach this from a dialectical perspective: as we saw, Freud already dedicated attention to ego functions. The development of the structural model caused him to take an ever-increasing interest in the relations between the individual and their external environment. And in Freud's final years, the ego came to occupy more of his interest, at the expense of the drives and internal reality (Govrin, 2004). Even in his therapeutic work, Freud emphasized adaptive behavior and included behavioral techniques (Freud, 1919b; Walter & Galston, 1946). But learning theory and a foregrounding of external reality were presented as "other" to psychoanalysis, and behaviorism (later on CBT) was criticized on the grounds of its narrow notion of the human condition, focusing as it does only on learning and information processing while failing to register human complexity (Miltone, 2001). It seems that learning abilities and adjustment to the external environment received less attention in psychoanalytic theory due to its need to maintain a separate and distinct identity. Psychoanalysis is often considered to be an isolationist approach, while the other functions to define and sustain self-definition and the values of the approach (Sampson, 1993).

From a dialectical point of view, psychoanalysis's criticism of learning theory and behaviorism is a negation of part of itself (adaptive behavior as we saw earlier), which then is externalized toward the other (in the shape of learning and later on information processing) for the purpose of isolating, bringing into focus its own identity. Ego psychology's emphasis on learning abilities, cognition, and adjustment, as functions of the ego itself, is the negation of this negated self-part through a sublation. This sublation simultaneously rejects and preserves something of the component; this was done in a way that does not repeat or is not identical to the original component as it first emerged in psychoanalysis (behavior and cognition now can be free from conflict and constitutes an initial development). At the same time, it is not the same as the first negation as it was seen in CBT (behavior or cognition does not meet a single component in theory and it is a part of the structural and topographical model in psychoanalysis). Ego psychology, in reincorporating these components, intended to broaden psychoanalytic theory so it would come to include those functions. Ego psychology, thus, created a knowledge structure with a "unity of identity and difference," which, while developing from its own otherness, remains faithful to psychoanalysis tradition.

Hartmann's elaboration of the ego in the structural theory remains relevant and has a contemporary value (Bornstein, 2022). Schafer (1999) sees Hartmann as Freud's metapsychology's most significant systematizer and mid-century modernizer. He presents him as a transitional figure in that he is the one who opened the gates of traditional Freudian psychoanalysis to object-relations thinking. According to Schafer, he did so by the central emphasis he put on adaptation while still committed to drive theory, metapsychology, and structural theory.

Beck's Cognitive Theory

As described, the beginnings of the CBT approach, with the first behavioral change and formation methods, can be found in behaviorism and learning theories. At this early stage of development, CBT, in contrast to psychoanalysis, focused on observed, measurable behavior that is subject to change using learning principles. Setting aside the psychoanalytic "psyche," behaviorism put human behavior at the center of its concern. Behaviorism rejected the idea that human behavior is the outcome of mental events, and this anti-mentalism became one of its major hallmarks (Govrin, 2015). It offered more straightforward, convincing explanations to some of the psychopathologies clinicians encountered. It consciously avoided vague, scientifically ungrounded terminology in response to the period's dominant psychoanalytic theories. Conceptualizations typical at this stage in its development tended to foreground the stimulus-response (input-output) schema (Hayes, 2004).

However, the simple association between stimulus and response which learning theory explained, beyond a mechanistic theoretical and therapeutic approach, did not relate to the complexities of human feeling, thought, and behavior. Against this background, the cognitive approach began to evolve in the 1960s by casting more light on the mediating factors between stimulus and response (cognition). Aaron Beck (1967, 1976) was the major representative of this development. He drew attention to patients' dysfunctional beliefs, seeking to gain insight into the features of irrational cognitions, find ways to change or adjust them, and thus influence both emotions and behavior (Hayes, 2004). Some main behaviorist components – its emphasis on exposure and acquisition of skills – remained part of the therapeutic protocols, but techniques for identifying, adjusting, and replacing nonrational cognitions, nonadaptive thinking patterns, and pathological schemes were added. Thus, on the one hand, the scientific tradition and the association between event and response stayed in place, therapy went on relying on protocols, and symptomatic change continued to be at the focus of work. On the other hand, human cognition entered the picture as a mediating factor.

This development did not happen in a vacuum, sprouting only from within the approach itself. It originated in an intersubjective context; Beck himself had started as a psychoanalyst, a direction he abandoned when his research on depression failed to confirm the assumption that depression was a form of internalized hostility, as suggested by Freud's motivational theory. Thus, the cognitive theory he formulated began with depression (1963, 1964) and sought to distinguish itself from psychoanalysis which ignored cognitive factors in its conceptualization of depression. Rejecting some key psychoanalytic terms, Beck proposed explaining depressive symptomatology from a cognitive perspective as an erroneous interpretation of events resulting from the activation of negative representations of self, world, and future (the cognitive triad).

Looking closely at patients' present problems rather than addressing past traumas, Beck tended to analyze directly accessible psychological experiences rather than the unconscious. Beck argued that there is a range of automatic thoughts occurring spontaneously and frequently in the margins of consciousness. They produce an immediate interpretation of the situation at hand. These automatic thoughts are distinguished from the ordinary flow of thoughts observed in reflective thinking or free association. Automatic thoughts originate in the deeper cognitive structures that constitute fundamental schemes or beliefs that store general and typical features of a stimulus, idea, or experience, and serve to organize new information meaningfully. These schemes are acquired early on in the individual's development. Thus, they come to function as filters when the present is processed (Knapp & Beck, 2008).

On the face of it, Beck could be understood as having rejected psychoanalytical theory's motivational model along with its conceptual, discursive domain, developing instead his rational cognitive model. But, on closer consideration, Rosner (2012), who researches Beck's writings, including private handwriting, argues that Beck was clearly influenced by the ego psychology of the 1950s and 1960s. She illustrates this by describing how Beck's schema development emerged from the structure of the "double wish," which derives from psychoanalytic conceptualizations. She argues that Beck's primitive cognitions and rational skills are analogous to the id and the ego, respectively. She claims that Beck first created a psychodynamic wish structure only after he drew an identical bipolar cognitive structure in his early works in the 1960s. Then he reached the schema structure which he published in his writings.

At a later stage in his writing, Beck acknowledges this influence (Beck, 1993; Knapp & Beck, 2008). He mentions that even though cognitive theory is generally known to have sprung from behavioral theory, it was influenced by, and reacted to, psychoanalytic ideas, especially those relating to the notion of primary processes (outside the range of consciousness, based on fantasies and desires) and secondary ones (consciously accessible, and based on principles aligned with objective reality). Beck initially identified himself as a neo-analyst, like Alfred Adler, Karen Horney, Otto Rank, and Harry Sullivan. They made a point of relating to and making sense of the patient's conscious experience and referring to the meaning patients attach to their life events. As we saw, Hartmann saw reason as the main component in human activity, and the irrational, to him, was of marginal importance, with its principal use in casting a light on rationality or as an obstacle to it. The ego, in this process, is seen as what can bring the individual closer to a correct, mature, and objective view of reality (Govrin, 2004). And so, this emphasis on cognition is, in part, a transformed element of the psychoanalytic tradition, which pays attention to intrapsychic processes.

However, this attention to cognition already existed in the behavioral approach (Wolpe, 1980). Arguably, since the latter approach emerged as a reaction against psychoanalysis, this element was negated and excluded, becoming alienated and identified with the psychoanalytic approach to provide an alternative and distinct identity. It is customary to think that the approach defines itself by contrast with other therapeutic streams (Safran & Messer, 1997).

From a dialectical point of view, the cognitive approach emerged from the behavioral approach, and from the absence of intrapsychic process. The cognitive approach sought to remain faithful to the behavioral approach but, by reference to information processing, to supply a simple answer to the intrapsychic complexities the psychoanalytic approach was looking at. This was attempted by rejecting the principle of the unconscious while embracing the principle of the mental (which the behavioral approach had rejected in its attempt to distinguish itself from psychoanalysis). Here we observe a dialectical process in action: the negation of a part that was previously negated, rejected, and alienated (the mental) is, again, negated at a later point in time. This does not restore the original identity nor its negation (in this case, the psychoanalytic unconscious), but leads to a complex idea that includes a unity of identity and difference (CBT's cognition).

Recent Developments

Due to the intensity and prevalence of personality disorders, later developments in the approaches led to far-reaching changes in their traditional approaches. However, the innovations stayed faithful to their respective roots. There is the development of schema therapy within the CBT approach, on the one hand, and MBT within the psychoanalytic approach, on the other. We will now demonstrate how these represent the DI process.

Schema therapy (Young, 1990; Young, Klosko & Weishaar, 2003) looks at the schemas a patient develops in response to early life circumstances, their innate temperament, and meaningful early relationships. According to this approach, these schemas affect an individual's way of seeing the world and acting in it, which then predisposes them to return to and repeat these same conditions in the present. Where basic needs were met sufficiently well, positive schemas develop, which do not result in suffering or distress. Insufficiently met needs, by contrast, are likely to trigger nonadaptive schemas (Rafaeli, Bernstein & Young, 2010).

This model relies significantly on Beck's cognitive theory, which introduced the notion of the basic schema. Beck had from early on considered schemas as the product of personal experience and the outcome of identification with significant others, and vice versa, of how the individual was being perceived by those significant others, in early development (Knapp & Beck, 2008). However, these observations about the developmental model of the schema did not feature centrally in his theory and practice. The focus was on the factors that maintain the schema. The developmental model and the influence of significant others were set aside as CBT evolved into a distinct entity and an alternative to psychoanalysis.

In view of the need for treatment of borderline personality disorder, Young and his collaborators elaborated the schema to include universal emotional needs, diverse self-states (modes), and coping styles. They gave special attention to past and present interpersonal relations, the development of current symptoms, and the therapist-patient relationship. In this case, Young et al. acknowledge integrating elements from attachment and object relations theories, gestalt and experiential therapies. At the same time, they continued to identify themselves as CBT therapists, rejecting psychoanalytic terminology and the concept of the unconscious, the model of the drives, and the resulting conflicts. For example, when they speak of schemas and coping responses being triggered unconsciously, it is only in the sense that they represent largely automatic reactions that occur without conscious awareness (Rafaeli, Bernstein & Young, 2010). The theory broadens Beck's cognitive theory and his concept of schema.

Here we also observe a dialectical process in action. First, cognitive theory negates a self-part that undergoes alienation in psychoanalysis (the developmental model and the influence of significant others are set aside). In this way, the approach maintains its distinctiveness and remains faithful to the core principles of CBT. Later, when a lacuna arises (treatment in personality disorders), the discipline negates this primary negation and re-internalizes the alienated self-component. This element does not restore the original identity (Beck's basic schema as the product of personal experience) nor its negation (the psychoanalytic concepts of unconscious object relations). As a result of a sublation, a complex idea is formed that encompasses identity and difference, introducing theoretical and practical development. Sublation as a movement of dialectical development rejects some aspects, on the one hand, and conserves fundamental content, on the other. Due to this, the concept continues to develop. This sublated concept of schema now emphasizes not only its development and the relationship with others that influences it, but also related concepts such as universal emotional needs, self-states (modes), and coping styles, further elaborating the schema concept. We can see how development continues to follow tradition's core principles and expands them within itself. Nevertheless, this process requires the other approach to make this development possible.

Another recent development, MBT (Bateman & Fonagy, 2004a, 2004b, 2006), brings together both classical (e.g., Winnicott) and contemporary (e.g., relational psychotherapy) psychoanalytic theories, on the one hand, and empirical approaches in the domain of developmental psychology (Bowlby's attachment theory) or cognitive psychology (ToM, Baron-Cohen's Theory of Mind), on the other.

This approach works on the assumption that, from infancy, we intuitively generate preconceptions and implicit mental explanations with regard to behaviors.

Mentalization includes the ability to think about our own thoughts, beliefs, feelings, and wishes, as well as those of others, and to understand that these internal events affect our own and other people's actions in many different ways. This approach emphasizes the development of the individual's ability to engage in mentalization rather than enhancing insight using an interpretation of the transference. For this purpose, the therapist encourages the patient to understand things differently and from various perspectives.

Those who developed this approach identify themselves as psychoanalysts and refer to Winnicott's and Bowlby's theories. But it seems, nevertheless, that some element originating in CBT theory has become incorporated into their model. In this case, too, dialectics is a productive way of approaching this development: Bateman and Fonagy argue that psychoanalysis has always addressed itself to the rehabilitation of the ability to mentalize in the sense that it aimed to enable patients to think and reflect on their behavior and to take an interest in their own and others' consciousness. The concept of mentalization is linked to that of insight. Mentalizing highlights the process by focusing on mental activity, while insight emphasizes the content (Allen, 2006).

While psychoanalysis first rejected cognition and processes of thought and thinking about thinking as extraneous, at this point in time the element of cognition returns in a different form (not in the original form in psychoanalysis as secondary processes, and not in its negation in the CBT approach; cognition as a mediating factor by introducing the schema). Here the cognitive component emerges naturally, as an integral part of psychoanalysis, and fits in with developmental theory, psychopathology, and therapeutic practice. While the new approach highlights thought processes, it continues to reject behavioral interventions and avows its principal interest in the patient's consciousness (its focus, that is, remains on the intrapsychic). And so, sublation produces a new knowledge structure (here mentalization) that preserves a dialectic tension in the identity of the approach and its body of knowledge.

Later developments in theories tend to recognize the influence of elements foreign to the theory. At the same time, even in these cases, loyalty to the mother school remains while distinguishing from the other school of thought. It seems that therapists are constantly exposed to ideas from other theories. They consciously and unconsciously incorporate elements from other therapies to which they have been exposed. Sometimes the assimilation is done consciously and while acknowledging the acceptance of the element as foreign, as in a model of integrative assimilation (Norcross & Alexander, 2019). In these cases, it is integrated with conscious intention and openness. Sometimes, the clash between an established therapeutic school and a new foreign component presents a unique challenge for those who do not support integration. In these situations, the newly imported concept can undergo a process of conversion that involves the "discovery" of its roots in the incorporating theory so that it can be presented as an integral part of that theory. This process is called "integration by conversion" (Govrin, 2016) and includes a conscious denial of integration.

Late developments acknowledge foreign components' influence as in integrative assimilation. At the same time, they also maintain that these ideas are an extension of the "mother theory" concepts. The dialectical process can help here as well. In our opinion, DI as an internal and unconscious developmental process can soften the opposition to those who oppose integration or feel the need to declare allegiance to the mother theory. We will discuss this in the following section.

Future Applications

We have introduced DI to articulate a new perspective on integration between psychotherapeutic approaches, and especially on the interactions between psychoanalysis and CBT. We have proposed, referring to Hegel's philosophy, to see these main psychotherapeutic approaches rather than self-enclosed totalities, static bodies of knowledge, as the dynamic product of a process of DI. Here reality is driven by the mutual conditioning between two perspectives, each taking shape in its encounter with the other. It is in this reciprocity that interdependence generates the totality of each as a unity in its own right, for neither of them can attain significance from within itself without referring to its otherness.

From a dialectical perspective, innovations must always emerge from tradition. What is new must be seen as a link in an existing chain, a natural development in an existing body of knowledge – in this case, a well-established and grounded therapeutic tradition. But at the same time, all development involves an element of otherness and strangeness – an element that is not simply extraneous to the tradition but also part and parcel of it.

Hegel's dialectics enriches our thinking about integration by overcoming the struggle with an extraneous otherness. This move is achieved neither by one side prevailing over the other nor by mutual agreement or compromise, and not by some third combination external to both. Instead, DI means recognition and containment of otherness and foreignness as such.

Kristeva (1991) elaborates on our ability to accept modes of otherness and the process whereby this ability matures into a relationship that does not erase otherness but in which it exists alongside our self-identification. Accepting the otherness within ourselves, she argues, will also allow us to accept the external other: "... The foreigner comes in when the consciousness of my difference arises, and he disappears when we all acknowledge ourselves as foreigners ..." (p. 1).

We would like to conclude by proposing Kristeva's argument that the ability of each approach to see the foreignness within it and itself as a foreigner can remove the threat of otherness and lead to an open position toward the other approach. This position may supply to those who are loyal to one approach, the rare distance from which the possibility of openness to the other arises, and along with it the ability to imagine and to think, to grow and change within themselves. For, as Hegel's dialectics show, though the difference and disjunction between approaches result in alienation, they equally lead to development. For Hegel, humankind distinguishes itself exactly by not only operating as a negating (and negated) power but being equipped with the rational and mental capacities necessary to cope with the destruction and anxiety of the negative and transform it for the sake of self-creation.

References

Allen, J.G. (2006) Mentalizing in practice. In: Allen, J. G. & Fonagy, P. (eds), *The Handbook of Mentalization-based Treatment* (pp. 3–30). Chichester, West Sussex: John Wiley & Sons.

Bateman, A.W. & Fonagy, P. (2004a) Mentalization-based treatment of BPD. *Journal of Personality Disorders* 18: 36–51.

Bateman, A.W. & Fonagy, P. (2004b) *Psychotherapy for Borderline Personality Disorder: Mentalization-based Treatment*. New York: Oxford University Press.

Bateman, A.W. & Fonagy, P. (2006) *Mentalization-based Treatment for Borderline Personality Disorder: A Practical Guide*. New York: Oxford University Press.

Beck, A.T. (1963) Thinking and depression: I. Idiosyncratic content and cognitive distortions. *Archives of General Psychiatry* 9: 324–33.

Beck, A.T. (1964) Thinking and depression: II. Theory and therapy. *Archives of General Psychiatry* 10: 561–71.

Beck, A.T. (1967) *Depression: Clinical, Experimental and Theoretical Aspects*. New York: Harper & Row.

Beck, A.T. (1976) *Cognitive Therapy and the Emotional Disorders*. New York: International Universities Press.

Beck, A.T. (1993) Cognitive therapy: Past, present and future. *Journal of Consulting and Clinical Psychology* 62(2): 194–8.

Blass, R.B. (2010a) Affirming 'That's not psychoanalysis!' On the value of the politically incorrect act of defining the field. *International Journal of Psychoanalysis* 91: 81–99.

Blass, R.B. (2010b) How does psychoanalytic practice differ from psychotherapy? The implications of the difference for the development of psychoanalytic training and practice: An introduction to 'Distinguishing Psychoanalysis from Psychotherapy'. *International Journal of Psychoanalysis* 91: 15–21.

Bornstein, M. (2022) Psychoanalysis, Heinz Hartmann and me: Pursuit of the love of life. *Psychoanalytic Inquiry* 42: 217–24.

Boswell, J.F., Sharpless, B.A., Greenberg, L.S., Heatherington, L., Huppert, J.D., Barber, J. P., et al. (2010) Schools of psychotherapy and the beginnings of a scientific approach. In: Barlow, D. H. (ed.), *The Oxford Handbook of Clinical Psychology* (pp. 98–127). Oxford: Oxford University Press.

Burke, V. (2005) Hegel's concept of mutual recognition: The limits of self-determination. *Philosophical Forum* 36(2): 213–20.

Cohen, R. S. & Wartofsky, M. W. (eds) (1984) *Hegel and the Sciences*, Volume 64. Dordrecht: Springer.

Edelstein, M.R., Kujoth, R.K. & Ramsay Steel, D. (2013) *Therapy Breakthrough: Why Some Psychotherapies Work Better Than Others*. Chicago, IL: Open Court Publishing.

Freud, S. (1919a) The 'Uncanny'. In: *The Standard Edition of the Complete Psychological Works of Sigmund Freud*, Volume XVII (1917–1919): An Infantile Neurosis and Other Works (pp. 217–256). London: Hogarth Press.

Freud, S. (1919b) Ways of the psychoanalytical therapy. In: Berman, E. & Rolnik, E. J. (eds), *Psychoanalytic Treatment* (Rolnik, E.J. trans.) (pp. 129–35). Tel-Aviv: Am-Oved, 2003.

Freud, S. (1923) The Ego and the Id. In: Strachey, J. et al. (trans.), *The Standard Edition of the Complete Psychological Works of Sigmund Freud*, Volume XIX. London: Hogarth Press.

Govrin, A. (2004) *Between Abstinence and Seduction—The Philosophy of American psychoanalysis*. Tel-Aviv: Dvir.

Govrin, A. (2015) *Conservative and radical Perspectives on Psychoanalytic Knowledge: The Fascinated and the Disenchanted*. London: Routledge.

Govrin, A. (2016) Blurring the threat of 'otherness': Integration by conversion in psychoanalysis and CBT. *Journal of Psychotherapy Integration* 26(1): 78–90.

Hartmann, H. (1939) *Ego Psychology and the Problem of Adaptation*. New York: International Universities Press, 1958.

Hartmann, H. (1964) *Essays on Ego Psychology*. New York: International Universities Press.

Hayes, S.C. (2004) Acceptance and commitment therapy and the new behavior therapies: Mindfulness, acceptance, and relationship. In: Hayes, S. C., Follette, V. M. & Linehan, M. (eds), *Mindfulness and Acceptance: Expanding the Cognitive-behavioral Tradition*. New York: Guilford Press.

Hegel, G.W.F. (2018) *The Phenomenology of Spirit* (Inwood, M. trans.). Oxford: Oxford University Press, 1807.

Kenan, A.M. (2019) The return of the subject to himself: Mutual recognition and projective identification. In: Govrin, A. (ed.), *Couch and Culture—Psychoanalysis Through Literature, Philosophy and Society* (pp. 263–302). Tel Aviv: Resling.

Klein, Y. (1978) The Dialectic of the Master and the Slave. Interpretation of a chapter from Hegel's *'Phenomenology of the Spirit'*. Tel Aviv: Am Oved.

Knapp, P. & Beck, A.T. (2008) Cognitive therapy: Foundations, conceptual models, applications and research. *Brazilian Journal of Psychiatry* 30: s54–64.

Knowles, D.R. (1985) Recent work on Hegel (book review). *The Philosophical Quarterly* 35(139): 199–204.

Kristeva, J. (1991) *Strangers to Ourselves*. New York: Columbia University Press, 1991.

Kubacki, S.R. & Chase, M. (1998) Comparing values and methods in psychodynamic and cognitive-behavioral therapy: Commonalities and differences. *Journal of Psychotherapy Integration* 8(1): 1–25.

Migone, P. (2011) Letter to the Editors On: The definition of psychoanalysis. *International Journal of Psychoanalysis* 92: 1315–17.

Mills, J. (2012) *The Unconscious Abyss: Hegel's Anticipation of Psychoanalysis*. Albany, NY: SUNY Press.

Miltone, J. (2001) Psychoanalysis and cognitive behavior therapy—Rival paradigms or common ground? *International Journal of Psychoanalysis* 82: 431–46.

Mitchell, S.A. & Black, M.J. (1995) *Freud and Beyond: A History of Modern Psychoanalytic Thought*. New York: Basic Books.

Norcross, J.C. & Alexander, E.F. (2019) A primer on psychotherapy integration. In: Norcross, J. C. & Goldfried, M. R. (eds), *Handbook of Psychotherapy Integration* (pp. 3–27). New York: Oxford University Press.

Peri Herzovich, Y. & Govrin, A. (2021) Psychoanalysis and CBT: From rivalry to hospitality in psychotherapy integration. *British Journal of Psychotherapy* 37: 244–62.

Rafaeli, E., Bernstein, D.P. & Young, J. (2010) *Schema Therapy: Distinctive Features*. London and New York: Routledge.

Rosner, R.I. (2012) Aaron T. Beck's drawings and the psychoanalytic origin story of cognitive therapy. *History of Psychology* 15(1): 1–43.

Safran, J.D. & Messer, S.B. (1997) Psychotherapy integration: A postmodern critique. *Clinical Psychology: Science & Practice* 4: 140–52.

Sampson, E.E. (1993) *Celebrating the Other: A Dialogic Account of Human Nature*. Boulder, CO: Westview Press.

Schafer, R. (1999) Recentering psychoanalysis: From Heinz Hartmann to the contemporary British Kleinians. *Psychoanalytic Psychology* 16: 339–54.

Skinner, B.F. (1953) *Science and Human Behavior*. New York: Macmillan.

Thagard, P. (1982) Hegel, science, and set theory. *Erkenntnis* 18: 397–410.

Tryon, W.W. (1986) The convergence of cognitive behaviorism and ego-psychology. *Theoretical & Philosophical Psychology* 6(2): 90–7.

Walter, B. & Galston, J.A. (1946) *Theme and Variations: An Autobiography*. New York: A. A. Knopf.

Wolpe, J. (1969) *The Practice of Behavior Therapy*. New York: Pergamon Press.

Wolpe, J. (1980) Cognitive behavior: A reply to three commentaries. *American Psychologist* 35(1): 112–14.

Yovel, Y. (1975) Hegel on reason, actuality and philosophical discourse. *Iyyun: The Jerusalem Philosophical Quarterly* July: 59–115.

Yovel, Y. (2005) Introduction. In: Hegel, G.W F., *Hegel's Preface to The Phenomenology of Spirit* (pp. 1–62). Princeton, NJ: Princeton University Press.

Young, J.E. (1990) *Cognitive Therapy for Personality Disorders: A Schema-focused Approach*. Sarasota, FL: Professional Resource Exchange.

Young, J.E., Klosko, J.S. & Weishaar, M.E. (2003) *Schema Therapy: A Practitioner's Guide*. New York: Guilford Press.

Chapter 4

Psychoanalysis and Interdisciplinarity with Nonanalytic Psychotherapeutic Approaches Through the Prism of Dialectics

Yael Peri Herzovich and Aner Govrin

In this chapter, we seek to broaden the perspective on psychoanalytic development through the lens of Hegelian dialectics – not solely in relation to cognitive-behavioral therapy (CBT) but in its encounters with various other disciplines as well.

Psychoanalysis, in its purist mainstream sense, tends to be considered as an isolationist discipline that steers clear of interdisciplinary connections with other psychotherapies. Its drive for purity does not open up to influences that cast as alien and a threat to its core principles. We refer to Hegelian dialectics in an attempt to offer an alternative approach to interdisciplinarity in clinical psychoanalysis. Psychoanalysis entertains a complex dialectical relationship with the major theories it opposes. In this dynamic, psychoanalysis begins by negating the non-psychoanalytic theory as a part of self-negation (Hegel calls this phase self-alienation). But in its own process of growth, it negates this negation and reabsorbs the alienated self part. Reabsorbing the negated component, psychoanalysis does not revert to its original identity but becomes sublated into a different, more complex idea. In this epistemological process, psychoanalysis deals with its own practical and theoretical anomalies and lacunas. We will illustrate this process using three central developments in the history of psychoanalysis: empathy in self psychology (connection with Rogers's humanist psychology), short-term dynamic psychotherapy (STDP; connection with short, intensive therapies), and mentalization-based psychotherapy (connection with CBTs). In all of these cases, psychoanalysis integrates components it previously opposed and changes these components to their own, specific characteristics. We address the epistemological shifts in the scientific status of psychoanalysis and show their connection to dialectics. Finally, we conclude that dialectical development is what allows psychoanalysis to remain relevant and up to date, to be open to interdisciplinary influences without its identity and tradition coming under threat.

Psychoanalysis and the Extra-Analytic Other

In recent years, there were several attempts to characterize the evolution of psychoanalytic thought. Makari (2000) posits that contemporary psychoanalysis, with its numerous models of mind and psychopathology, includes both a far-reaching and

DOI: 10.4324/9781003608103-5

vital Kuhnian proto-science, as well as a historically deep practice of meanings and values. Makari believes that change in psychoanalysis is not uniform. Rather, some progress in psychoanalysis reflects the kinds of shifts Kuhn ascribed to a proto-science and change that propose a new net of meanings, an ethic, a way to live in the world. Govrin (2004) argues that shifts in epistemological assumptions have always accompanied significant ideological nodes in the history of psychoanalysis. In other words, the psychoanalytic therapeutic concepts have changed because the cultural and philosophical context of the world view has changed, mainly from positivism to postmodernism.

In this chapter, we would like to describe the evolution of psychoanalysis by using Hegel's dialectic process stages. But let us first clarify what we mean when using the broad term "psychoanalysis" and what we do not mean.

The field of psychoanalysis has gone through many theoretical evolutions since Freud's time, from an emphasis on the drives to ego psychology, object relations theory, and self psychology, and is currently preoccupied with postmodern perspectives and those focusing on relationality and intersubjectivity. Therefore, psychoanalysis is not (anymore) a "monolith" but includes within it a multitude of different positions. These include ones that seek to integrate psychoanalysis and other nonanalytic approaches (such as neuropsychoanalysis, infant research, and integration with CBT and other orientations). It is important to note that in this chapter, we use "psychoanalysis" in its purist mainstream sense by which the nucleus of the identity of psychoanalysis lies in the "understanding" of unconscious dynamics (Migone, 2011) and uncovering and understanding the (often unconscious) conflicts and early developmental experiences associated with the client's symptoms (Boswell et al., 2010). We are aware that many other forms of psychoanalysis are oriented toward integration and mutual influence with nonanalytic theories (they are usually heavily criticized by the "purists" [see, for example, Blass and Carmeli's (2007) criticism of neuropsychoanalysis, and Green's (2000) criticism against infant research]). We are also aware that in many contemporary psychoanalytic approaches, there is not that a rigid opposition between psychoanalysis and non-psychoanalysis, being themselves not considered psychoanalytic by classical or more conservative psychoanalysts (see, for example, the intersubjective or the relational tracks, etc.). However, we believe that mainstream psychoanalysis is still a dominant force, especially today when psychoanalysis needs to show its relevancy in a world that offers many other effective therapies. Furthermore, psychoanalysis still often defines itself by reference to what it is not, which means other psychotherapeutic schools.

This chapter will therefore concentrate on a specific phenomenon or trend within mainstream psychoanalysis that reflects itself within many psychodynamics clinicians (Govrin, 2015) – analyst's indifference to nonanalytic approaches. This is reflected by the following: (a) psychoanalysis flagship journals tend to be "purists" and to overlook important developments in other fields, and (b) training in many psychoanalytic institutes is essentially non-integrative. Cherry et al. (2020) conducted interviews with 69 graduates from the Columbia University Center for

Psychoanalytic Training and Research since 2003. It seems that the nonanalytic world had little if any place in their psychoanalytic education. Furthermore, one of the significant aims of training of the twenty first century is to show the advantage of psychoanalysis over other approaches. Fritsch and Winer (2020), in their propose "A Model of Psychoanalytic Education for the Twenty-First Century," write:

> Training the fertile fields of the 1950s had become the desert of the 2000s. A popular explanation was that we had lost cultural currency. We had been replaced both by new therapeutic approaches that promised greater benefits, faster and at a fraction of the price – CBT, DBT, Prozac – and by other sorts of mental and physical approaches: yoga, mindfulness training, EMDR.
>
> (p. 175)

(c) Case studies are almost exclusively pure psychoanalytic and rarely integrate other ideas from nonanalytic theories.

The indifference to nonanalytic theories is reflected by a dismissive approach, sometimes by criticism (Shedler, 2015; Westen et al., 2004) and most often by overlooking it. Govrin (2015) has explained the relative indifference of analysts to other theories by showing that analysts use narratives that are coherent all-encompassing and useful even when therapeutic failures occur. Alternative theories simply do not fit the coherence of the narrative and therefore are of no use. A Foucauldian perspective also sheds light on psychoanalysis's wholeness:

> Psychoanalysis is the term by which we designate one of the disciplines among the psychological and social sciences, a discipline that includes a taken-for-granted understanding of the human subject and a therapeutic technology for its management. The assemblage that comprises psychoanalysis as a discipline entails a particular discourse on human existence, a life-and identity-defining master narrative which articulates a specific form of the subject that is asserted to be natural, essential, ahistorical, and universal.
>
> (Milchman & Rosenberg, 2011, p.6)

Rejection to empirical findings and to new paradigms is widespread in science. Many post-positivist philosophers of science described scientist's resistance to change even in the face of contradicting findings. Cohen (1985), for example, writes:

> The desire to be an active part of a revolutionary movement is often in conflict with the natural reluctance of any scientist to jettison the set of accepted ideas on which he has made his way in the profession. New and revolutionary systems of science tend to be resisted rather than welcomed with open arms because every successful scientist has a vested intellectual, social, and even financial interest in maintaining the status quo.
>
> (p. 35)

In *The Origins of Modern Science*, Butterfield (1997) argued that "the most difficult mental act of all is to rearrange a familiar bundle of data, to look at it differently and escape from prevailing doctrine" (p. 106). He also writes that

> of all forms of mental activity, the most difficult to induce even in the minds of the young, who may be presumed not to have lost their flexibility, is the art of handling the same bundle of data as before but placing them in a new system of relations with one another by giving them a different framework.
>
> (p. 13)

While rejecting evidence and resistance to change are features characterizing science at the descriptive level of discourse, science must be open to new evidence and change at the prescriptive level.

Psychoanalysis (in the sense we use it here) tends to be considered an isolationist discipline that makes few interdisciplinary connections with other psychotherapies. There is a common belief that psychoanalysts interact almost exclusively with each other (Malcolm, 1982). By doing so, they deprive themselves of exposure to competing viewpoints and alternative perspectives that might enrich the psychoanalytic model (Bornstein, 2001). Training programs, major journals in the field, conferences, and the general psychoanalytic discourse invest little effort in nonanalytic clinical theories and the many possibilities the introduction of some of their ideas might hold. The approach surrounds itself with a faithful community of professionals who identify with it and often define themselves by contrast with other therapeutic streams (Safran & Messer, 1997). Many scholars who reflect on this phenomenon usually think that a therapist from another therapeutic persuasion is regarded as belonging to a foreign culture (Wachtel, 2010) and that the other functions to define and maintain self-definition and the values of the approach (Sampson, 1993). The distinction between us vs them helps to consolidate those who follow the method and give them political power (Sorenson, 2000).

Loyalists' main worry is that psychoanalysis, once exposed to another, alien direction, will not manage its own tradition's mainstay, like bringing the unconscious to consciousness. As a result, the profession, it is feared, may cave in before superficial, intense, and fast therapies (e.g., Blass [2010] and Berman [2010], response]. Psychoanalysis's motivation for maintaining the tradition's mainstay in therapeutic theory and practice consists of many reasons (some mentioned above). First, psychoanalysis is a theory and technique for treating psychological disorders; it deals with the relief of mental suffering. Its followers believe its ideas about what can count as an effective therapy (Wachtel, 2018). Second, it also involves economic competition over public resources, recognition, and prestige (Miltone, 2001; Shahar, 2011). Also, a fear of questioning identity and the wish to maintain a solid and robust identity is another reason why boundaries between schools are required (Peri Herzovich & Govrin, 2021).

Any object that threatens us must be an object which we already recognize as relevant to us, as being in some relation to us. Not everything outside us is experienced as a threat: an alternative psychotherapeutic approach may be perceived as a threat by psychoanalysis, where a new mathematical model won't. Kristeva (1991/1988) argued that what we consider foreign – which manifests as hatred of the other – includes a hidden aspect of our own identity. The difficulty we have in accepting the other, she believes, is the outcome of our inability to acknowledge our own subjective otherness. As a result, we experience those unlike us as a threat and need to keep them out. Kristeva refers to the Freudian unconscious in her description of the hatred of the stranger as a manifestation of the unconscious projection and rejection of uncontrollable drives or unprocessed parts. In his writing about the uncanny, Freud puts this as follows: "[...] for this uncanny is in reality nothing new or alien, but something which is familiar and old-established in the mind and which has become alienated from it only through the process of repression" (Freud, 1919, p. 241). And so what is alien and threatening are materials that have undergone repression and exclusion processes to be removed from ourselves. That is to say, there is both a process of repression and a process of externalization of self components, both of which are done unconsciously. The common result is that what I experience as a stranger and as an other is not only his or her own foreignness but actually a foreignness of myself. This is why, in this chapter, we argue that the alienness of non-psychoanalytic approaches, in addition to forming an external threat, also represents the threat from within.

In this chapter, we would like to add another aspect to the relations between mainstream psychoanalysis and nonanalytic theories to show the dialectic nature of their relations. We refer to Hegel's epistemology (epistemology as the study of knowledge) to show that psychoanalysis evolves dialectically by integrating or assimilating external influences like other bodies of knowledge that also represent reabsorbing alienated self parts.

Hegel was one of the first historical epistemologists. His dialectics is a general developmental theory of the subject, but it is particularly relevant to the development of knowledge. If we look at psychoanalysis's history through the lens of dialectics, we find that psychoanalysis's attitude to other therapeutic methods is more complicated than meets the eye. We perceive the quest for purity in psychoanalysis as a form of self-negation. Still, we believe it is only part of an entire dialectical process by which psychoanalysis does uniquely incorporate external components. While the dialectic process of affirmation of identity and becoming is unconscious, what is conscious is the consideration of other approaches as alien and extraneous to the psychoanalytic field.

Although we cannot give a complete representation of Hegel's dialectic, it is possible to capture some of the dialectics' essential features that will shed new light on the intricate relations between psychoanalysis and other psychotherapies. According to Mills (2012), what is central to Hegel's overall philosophy is the notion of process, a thesis that has direct implications for the development of psychoanalysis. But "One does not have to espouse Hegel's entire philosophical system, which is neither necessary nor desirable, in order to appreciate the dialectic and its application to psychoanalysis and contemporary modes of thought" (p. 188).

Dialectic development in psychoanalysis occurs when an initial component of it undergoes *negation*, is rejected, and is projected onto the therapeutic other (Hegel calls this phase self-alienation). Negation can take the form of criticism or total disregard, and it serves to preserve the clear identity of the theory. Over time, however, when the approach fails to offer a sufficient response to clinical challenges, *a negation of the negation*, the next step in the dialectical process, takes place. The previously cast-off, negated part is restored to the theory to deal with the perceived lack. However, as it performs this negation, it dialectically produces a synthesis with the negated component on a higher level, namely by including it, theoretically and/ or practically, in a new guise. When this negated element is incorporated in the mainstream, by negating its negation, it does not retain its original identity. This is where Hegel's notion of *Aufhebung* or sublation comes in: the newly integrated element produces a more complex and different idea. While sublation negates and rejects the negated component, it also preserves that component's essence, thereby raising psychoanalysis to a higher level. In this manner, we can describe how psychoanalysis develops in a dialectic process that tends to perfection, a stage which Hegel called Absolute Knowledge.

Hegel's idealism seeks to offer a total and absolute account of the development of the subject and of knowledge that was appropriate to his times. In our postmodern reality, such total idealist theories have become controversial. We suggest focusing on Hegel's description of the dialectical dynamic through which both subject and knowledge emerge, taking an epistemic perspective. This, we believe, yields a new way of looking at the history of psychoanalytic thinking. Considering this history as dialectical, we perceive it as interdisciplinary in essence. Such an approach resolves the tension in psychoanalysis's attitude to other psychotherapeutic disciplines because it shows how it needs them to constitute its own distinct and separate identity.

It is important to note that every human endeavor might be represented as interdisciplinary in essence. However, among different disciplines, psychoanalysis's inclination toward interdisciplinary is remarkable since it touches on so many different aspects: science, hermeneutics, biology, development, brain research, philosophy, art, and humanities. Still, the interdisciplinary relationship between psychoanalysis and other nonanalytic psychotherapeutic approaches has not been sufficiently explored.

In the first part of this chapter, we present Hegelian dialectics to explain how scientific knowledge develops. We shall limit ourselves to some of its central and important concepts. In the second part, we put these concepts to use in describing three major developments in psychoanalysis: the introduction and incorporation of self psychology, including the notion of empathy (by way of linking with Rogers's humanist psychology), STDP (by way of linking with intensive therapies), and mentalization-based therapy (by way of linking with cognitive-behavioral psychology). In the third part, we refer to the scientific status of psychoanalysis and shifts in epistemological positioning. In the concluding section, we will discuss the importance of dialectic processes in maintaining psychoanalysis's vitality.

It is important to note that Hegel's dialectical process can describe the evolution of all psychotherapies such as CBT, Gestalt therapy, family systems theory, and emotion-focused therapy. Indeed, Hegel takes dialectic to be a general theory of development. Hegel (1892b) says that "wherever there is movement, wherever there is life, wherever anything is carried into effect in the actual world, there Dialectic is at work." (p. 148). Govrin (2016) described how CBT endorsed mindfulness, a spiritual Zen practice, and incorporated it within its rational scientific worldview by a process called "integration through conversion."

As in psychoanalysis, a similar diversity could be found in other psychotherapy movements, too (Castiglioni & Corradini, 2011). For example, there are two strands partially opposed to each other within the systemic movement: (a) the "Philadelphia School," which since the 1960s has tried to combine the systemic model with psychoanalytic concepts; (b) the "system purists" who reject all contaminations with "intrapsychic" models, in particular psychoanalysis, to focus – in an entirely relational perspective – on the analysis of pathogenic communicative models (cf. Gurman & Kniskern, 1981–1991). However, we believe psychoanalysis is perhaps the most interesting case to demonstrate its evolution by the dialectic process because no other psychotherapeutic school was characterized by so much negation, dismissal, and resistance to change, whether through bitter controversies between new and old psychoanalytic schools (for the Freud-Klein controversies, see Steiner, 1991) or through dismissing nonanalytic theories. Nearly all nonanalytic psychotherapies such as client-centered therapy, family systems therapy, Gestalt therapy, and CBT evolved through negation of psychoanalysis principles, and it can be demonstrated that through a dialectic process how the negated elements have been incorporated into these systems later in a new guise, but this deserves a separate paper.

Hegel's Method

Though Hegel's thought is dense and detailed, it is possible to describe the dialectics' main thesis quite concisely. According to Thagard (1982), Hegel elaborated his dialectics concerning consciousness in his *The Phenomenology of Spirit* (Hegel, 2018/1807) and in relation to history in his *Philosophy of History* (Hegel, 1956/1837), and more specifically to the history of philosophy in *Lectures on the History of Philosophy* (Hegel, 1892a), and to the logical categories in *Science of Logic* (Hegel, 1969/1812). In the first of these, Hegel elaborates how human consciousness emerges from containing only the most primitive knowledge to having the capacity to attain absolute knowledge. His logical categories describe how a "notion" evolves from the most primitive category – Being – to the overarching category of the Absolute Idea. Every process, Hegel argues, has the same structure. Thus, about consciousness, he writes: "the development of this object, like the development of all-natural and spiritual life, rests solely on the nature of the pure essentialities which constitute the content of logic" (Hegel, 1969/1812, p. 28). Still, one can form a particularly clear understanding of how Hegel's dialectics construes the growth of scientific knowledge from the dialectics of the stages of consciousness, as they appear in *The Phenomenology of Spirit* (Hegel, 2018/1807), compared, for instance, to his pure dialectics of logic (in *Science of Logic* [Hegel, 1969/1812]): in the former, he foregrounds the human subject's development of knowledge. Our discussion, therefore, is especially relevant to the dialectics of consciousness described in the former text.

Below we will describe the dialectical process of the formation of the subject that also obtains for the process whereby knowledge is consolidated. That will be described after it as the development of a subject-like system.

Development of the Dialectics of Self-Consciousness

The Phenomenology of Spirit (Hegel, 2018/1807) describes the emergence of the subject, from a *consciousness* whose content is another object to *self-consciousness* – now the object of consciousness is its self. This process, for Hegel, requires another subject. It is in the encounter with the other and through mutual recognition that the two sides constitute themselves as self-conscious subjects.

Hegel begins by distinguishing between subject and object. While the object is a primary, simple given which operates according to the principle of self-identity (A=A), the subject is not a priori given and is never identical to itself. The subject constructs its identity and knowledge through a dialectical relationship between difference and identity. This happens in a three-stage, iterative, cyclic process: *identity, the negation of identity* and therefore difference, the *negation of difference* and therefore identity, and hence renewed identity. When the identity between two things is negated, difference, or opposition, between them emerges, and when this is followed by the negation of difference as opposition, identity is reestablished. But this third stage, the negation of the negation, does not take us back to where we began. It produces a new, more complex tier of identity. This new level of identity is of a higher order, and it goes by the name dialectical identity. Dialectical identity simultaneously retains the difference between the two terms it includes but also cancels it, allowing their identity (Levkovich, 2011).

A particular content's primary form is negated and canceled in every dialectical process while its fundamental meaning is maintained on a higher level of formalization and expression. This content, preserved as an element in the new condition, comes about through what Hegel called *sublation* (the German word *Aufhebung* literally refers to negation or cancellation and elevation and a movement upward and ahead [Yovel, 2001]). Each new stage sublates the one before it and replaces it. So sublation is a type of dialectic development including three moments: the negation or cancellation of a given form, retention of the fundamental content, and raising this content to a higher level of expression. Certain components are rejected in this process as essential components are accepted and preserved. Sublation retains and preserves, while also criticizing earlier forms of thinking and discarding them. It is always a qualitative renewal process, which raises the subject to a higher ontological and epistemological level. This is a dialectical, not a simple linear, analytical mode of development (Yovel, 1975).

Having described dialectical identity and the process of dialectical development, the next question to be addressed is the position of the other. In Hegel's view, the subject's identity emerges through self-alienation, whereby it becomes other than itself (negation). This implies that what is perceived as other always includes a negated part of the primary identity. It is by returning to the self from this otherness (negation of the negation) – in which the self has recognized the other and hence his own internal otherness – that consciousness can come to recognize itself, to evolve into self-consciousness attaining its own realization.

It must be stressed that the other is an actual other and not just the internal otherness of consciousness. On the one hand, it is not the self; it is, on the other, a moment of self-consciousness. Consciousness needs another consciousness to know itself. This can be explained as follows:

Subjective identity, as said, must be considered as an act of self-identification performed by reference to the other, something which is achieved at the end of a process. It is not identical to itself from the start and only approaches itself through repeated negations of its opposites, through the negation of the negation. Again, dialectical development takes off with the act of negation of a part of itself. The subject casts off this part and identifies it in the other who is experienced as foreign to it. When the dialectical process unfolds properly, the subject returns to itself through the negation of the negation.

The components of itself which it formerly negated are now identified as so-called *moments* of the self. For the subject to recognize these multiple moments as his own, and at the same time have a unifying pattern of himself, he needs the mediation of the other. This is because the realization of every being in nature is conditional on the existence of the two moments that constitute its full essence: a moment of plurality and a moment of unity. Human consciousness holds both these moments. It contains the essence of Being, yet it also is Being itself and in need of another consciousness that can have its own moments. Unable to validate itself, human consciousness turns to another who will provide its full realization, namely the moment of its plurality and the moment of its unity (Shalgi, 2009).

Self-consciousness, therefore, is possible only where it is reflected in another self-consciousness; the latter serves as the means whereby consciousness knows itself, or, in Hegel's own words: "Self-consciousness is in and for itself, when, and by the fact that it is in and for itself for another self-consciousness; that is, it is only as something recognized" (Hegel, 2018/1807, p. 76, s.178).

The Dialectical Development of the Subject-Like Structure

As said, Hegel's dialectics describes not only the emergence of the human subject but also that of subject-like structures. Dialectic logic traces the dynamic structure of mental structures insofar as they are subject-like structures, including the development of knowledge and science (Cohen & Wartofsky, 1984). The subject-like structure evolves through the other – in this case: other bodies of knowledge. Dialectical development is an iterative process that continues until the absolute realization of the subject or the body of knowledge (which constitutes self-consciousness), a condition Hegel calls the Spirit or Absolute Knowledge.

No subject-like structure features one simple and primary identity: its realization must be understood as an act of self-identification through otherness and the other. Whether we are dealing with a human entity or an entity of knowledge, both take the shape of a subject (having self-consciousness), which is never what it is right from the start and rather proceeds toward itself through its opposites: the plural and the other. A knowledge entity, therefore, comes about similarly as a subject through negation.

Negations do not take the process back to where it began: each act of negation institutes a different state of affairs (and consciousness). Earlier stages are not erased by negation: they are retained in the very texture of the next stage as a type of memory, expressing sublation. At each stage, the collapse of one position advances the process toward another position serving as a specific, even if temporary, response to the specific fault which came to light at the earlier stage and caused its collapse (such faults, in science, are called anomalies, lacunae, or unresolved problems). In this process, the entity of knowledge (or the subject-like structure) assumes various forms and contents that are retrospectively considered as expressions of its self. Thus, this is permanently becoming and does not exist in actuality, except for eventually, at the end of the process (if there is such a thing) when it is realized in the complete process and its result (Yovel, 2001).

So, for Hegel, a knowledge entity comes into being in the same manner as self-consciousness. As a subject-like structure, the concept of science refers to a knowledge entity or a system of cognition which, from being an opinion, has become an *episteme*. Scientificity, here, does not denote one or another domain of knowledge or expertise but a degree (the highest degree) of cognition that every domain of knowledge seeks to attain. For Hegel, science is the totality of its components. Developments in the body of knowledge, for him, constitute stages in the development of the Spirit. Rather than being judged as true or false, they must be considered in terms of more or less mature, with each given developmental stage including those that came before it.

So when a knowledge entity evolves into its realization as science, this does not take the shape of linear progress, but instead of dialectical movement, that is to say, a cyclic development of a subject-like structure, which negates its own point of departure and returns to it on a different level, through a process of mutual negations. This yields a stable system that, staying in constant motion, avoids fixation (Yovel, 2001).

Hegel's method, to conclude, describes the developmental totality of a system that retains all the fundamental achievements made in the process. The realization of absolute knowledge approaches itself through opposites and by means of negation: through plurality and otherness. Hence, this development requires an initial resistance of a body of knowledge to otherness, followed, later on, by recognizing other entities of knowledge that are relevant to itself and thereby recognizing itself for the sake of its ongoing development.

Hegel's dialectic is a general theory of scientific knowledge. It corresponds to many aspects of the post-positivist philosophy of science. According to Thagard (1982), "each stage of the dialectic bears the same sort of complex relation to the previous stage as a scientific theory does to its predecessor" (p. 397). According to Hegel, the self-development of the subject (or subject-like structures in this case) is dependent upon recognition by other subjects. Understanding the dynamics of Hegel's dialectical method may lead to a new understanding of the historical development of psychoanalysis, as interdisciplinary in essence, in the process of becoming. Below we will employ the above principles of Hegel's method to discuss how bodies of knowledge outside the psychoanalysis domain affect the latter's dialectical development as a distinct yet simultaneously interdisciplinary domain, a mode of development that is vital and indispensable to it.

The Dialectical Nature of the Interdisciplinary Encounter Between Psychoanalysis and Non-psychoanalytic Bodies of Knowledge

Here we illustrate the dialectical development of psychoanalysis in its encounter with non-psychoanalytic bodies of knowledge by looking at three important developments in psychoanalysis: Kohut's self psychology, STDP, and mentalization-based psychotherapy.

Kohut's Self Psychology

Kohut started to develop self psychology in the 1960s because of difficulties he and most other therapists were having in treating certain patients with so-called narcissistic disorders: issues concerning self-esteem, self-equilibrium, self-regulation, and patients' very core sense of being. Analysts usually addressed these demanding, frustrating, and frequently grandiose clients by interpreting their constant demands on the analyst as stemming from defenses against unconscious aggressive and sexual Oedipal feelings directed toward the analyst. These interpretations usually enraged or depressed these patients, leading analysts, beginning with Freud, to conclude that they could not be analyzed (Tobin, 1991).

Kohut's self psychology (Kohut, 1971, 1977, 1984) foregrounded the power of empathy. He believed that any attempt to understand a patient must have its beginnings in empathy, and he called for the existing psychoanalytic practice to incorporate this insight. In his first major published article, Kohut challenged traditional psychoanalytic practitioners. He announced that the psychoanalyst's job should consist of more than the passive contemplation of the patient's free associations and the subsequent analysis of their resistance. Kohut believed that only by imagining ourselves in the patient's place employing *vicarious introspection* can we bring to life unknown inner experiences. Unlike the mainstream psychoanalysis of his time, which focused on the transference, the unconscious, and recollection, Kohut proposed a method of *empathic validation*, enabling the therapist to validate the patient's description. Kohut rejected interpretation as psychoanalysis's exclusive tool and employed extended empathic interventions to confirm the patient's perception. It is the therapist's task, he believed, to give the patient a sense of the therapist's identification with her or his feelings and to show them their understanding. Any other psychotherapy is at risk of making the patient feel ununderstood, dealing a serious blow to their narcissism.

However, the notion of empathy had already come to be seen as part of Carl Rogers's humanistic method and considered a foreign element by psychoanalysis. Rogers (1942) had been treating patients by using empathy in the 1940s. Kohut and Rogers worked at Chicago University, and although the two never met, they knew about each other (Kahn & Rachman, 2000). The problem, however, was that Rogers had developed his therapy as an alternative to psychoanalysis. On its face, the two methods seemed to clash since psychoanalysis posited that the most important therapeutic process was uncovering the unconscious and insight based on interpretation, not on empathic validation.

Indeed, Kohut was critical of nonanalytic and non-interpretive psychotherapeutic counseling, such as the humanistic approach. He likened such psychotherapeutic methods to the work of a repairman who manages to get his old alarm clock to work. Knowing nothing about clocks, all he actually did was to clean it up and oil the internal mechanism (Kohut, 1978, p. 525).

Kohut faced a problem: Could he identify psychoanalysis with an approach which he rejected and criticized? His ideas, indeed, met with strong opposition to begin with. They were taken to clash with psychoanalysis's most fundamental assumptions. Kohut was accused of mocking Freud's core values, appropriating concepts, populism, superficiality, subjectivity, ignoring the unconscious's role, rejecting the scientific method, and turning psychoanalysis into a one-dimensional method (Brenner, 1968; Moses, 1988; Stein, 1979). And yet, part of the psychoanalytic community welcomed his ideas warmly (Menaker, 1978; Schwartz, 1978). As time went by, even the most conservative institutions came to include them in their training programs. Kohut's body of work has proven to have a tremendous impact on the clinical theory and practice of psychoanalysts over the last decades (Carr & Cortina, 2011).

We would like to argue that Kohut's eventual embrace by the psychoanalytic establishment resulted from a dialectical maneuver of self psychology. Empathy was not really foreign to psychoanalysis: Freud referred to it several times in his texts on the joke (Freud, 1905) and group psychology (Freud, 1921). That said, he never used empathy as a significant analytic tool. This may have been due to Freud's desire to cast psychoanalysis as a scientific body of knowledge. Rather than introducing Rogers's "alien" element of empathy, which the psychoanalytic community rejected, Kohut showed that the scientific tradition of psychoanalysis itself implied it. He believed that psychoanalysis could not do without empathy and that it, moreover, was already active in psychoanalytic practice. He showed that empathy cohered with psychoanalysis in its basic function of data collection for the improved understanding of the patient's unconscious dynamic (Kohut, 1959). Kohut (1975) argued that empathy, being a tool for data collection just like the microscope assists the physician to examine a patient's blood, confirmed the scientific nature of psychoanalysis. Meanwhile, to ensure the status of psychoanalysis's distinct, autonomous identity, he also criticized nonanalytic and non-interpretive forms of psychological counseling like humanistic psychotherapy (Kahn & Rachman, 2000).

We can then conclude that the component of subjective empathy (self), which was rejected and alienated (other), returned (self) following the negation of its negation, but – through sublation – rather than coming back in the very same form, it returned not as an emotive function but in a new, sublated form. In this process, the idea of empathy became part of psychoanalytic tradition, its definition of the unconscious, and scientificity. Kohut's simultaneous rejection of nonanalytic approaches made self- psychology's entrance into mainstream psychoanalysis possible. The distinction between them and us had been preserved, even though, *and because*, this development had been prompted by an encounter with an ostensibly foreign element. This tension between autonomy and dependence was vital in the emergence of psychoanalysis's dialectic identity and its development as a body of knowledge.

Short-Term Dynamic Psychotherapy

At the same time as Kohut was attempting to change the face of psychoanalysis by introducing the concept of empathy, another no less daring attempt to change the psychoanalytic landscape was underway: the introduction of STDP.

The spread in the course of the 1970s and 1980s, and even before, of competing forms of nonanalytic short intervention such as planned short-term therapy (an example of such nonanalytic new psychotherapies is Milton Erickson's brief and strategic model of psychotherapy (Erickson, 1954) and the strategic family therapy by Haley [1963]), which offered a written protocol and highly technical approach designed for brief treatments, was quite remarkable. Many of the new methods registered an achievement that gave them a distinct edge over psychoanalysis: Not only were they quicker and cheaper, but they were also supported by research that proved their efficacy (Lemma et al., 2010).

The originators of STDP looked beyond the psychoanalytic world and were willing to respond to these presented challenges. In the main, short-term therapy was developed during the 1980s and 1990s by several key psychoanalysts: Mann in Boston (Mann, 1973; Mann & Goldman, 1982), Malan in London (Malan, 1963, 1976), Sifneos in Boston (Sifneos, 1972, 1979), and Davanloo in Montreal (Davanloo, 1978, 1980). Additional founders include Donovan (1987), Gustafson (1984), Strupp and Binder (1984), and Luborsky (1984). These orthodox psychoanalysts were looking for solutions to needs that the classical approach failed to meet and sought to cope with its limitations (Mann & Goldman, 1982).

Short-term therapies seemed to breach all-important psychoanalytic assumptions at once: free associations were replaced by focused therapy; neutrality and evenly suspended attention – two fundamental analytical attitudes recommended by Freud (1912, 1915) – were substituted by therapists' active and directed interventions; the structural change was replaced by resolving a central conflict.

These changes raise the question of what elements of classical psychoanalysis we deem to be essential. How were psychoanalysts persuaded to try and resolve an Oedipus complex within the span of 15 meetings? How did they abandon free association for the sake of focused therapy? What made them become more directly involved, setting aside the pivotal psychoanalytic mode of therapeutic neutrality? These questions can be explained by means of Hegelian dialectics.

First, supporters of the new method pointed out the roots of the technique within the psychoanalytical tradition, particularly in its founder's works. Freud's early treatments were very short, compared not only to today's psychoanalysis but even in terms of today's dynamic short-term analysis. Freud met with Katarina (Freud & Breuer, 1955/1895) only once and yet regarded the meeting as a psychoanalytic session. Gustav Mahler's consultation with Freud was also limited to one session (Jones, 1955; Reik, 1960).

Second, supporters of the approach argued that there were no clashes between a time-bound therapeutic setting, and the psychoanalytic approach to the psyche, its theoretical model, and associated therapeutic techniques. They emphasized that STDP was more effective in achieving analytic objectives than long-term treatment. That is to say, using STDP is not merely a compromise imposed by necessity but rather a better implementation of classical treatment. Moreover, proponents of STDP strictly stuck to employing psychoanalytic terminology and jargon.

One of the most representative examples of STDP is Mann's (1973) *Time-Limited Psychotherapy*. Mann limited therapy to a series of 12 sessions following an initial assessment. The idea behind this was to turn time into an active psychoanalytic-therapeutic component. Termination, and hence the time limit, can serve as the main lever for the intensive, fast mobilization of processing and change. The time limit introduces the reality principle into the therapeutic space as opposed to the pleasure principle. This rallies the forces of the ego. Mann also argued that the therapeutic focus on a "main issue" (a problem the patient has been experiencing early on in their life) was a working principle that cohered with classical psychoanalysis. Mann did not seek to replace psychoanalysis; he intended to refine and develop it.

We witness how STDP restored elements to psychoanalysis that were initially negated. When the negation of elements like therapeutic focus, active position, and especially short term is negated, they do not return to their previous identity; through sublation, they become more complex and lead to theoretical development. The method becomes relevant and accessible to a larger population, including public mental health clinics that cannot offer long-term therapies. This would not have happened without dialectic development. Here the tension of the interdisciplinary encounter with the therapeutic other and the psychoanalytic tradition's organic growth allows for the mainstream to accept the new development.

Mentalization-Based Treatment

Another change in psychoanalysis occurred in the 1990s. Confronting intensified psychological problems and an access of personality disorders, psychoanalytic communities were prompted to introduce unprecedented change in their modes of treatment while also remaining loyal to the approach from which they had developed.

Mentalization-based treatment (MBT) emerged especially in the context of a growing need to address borderline disorder (according to the *Diagnostic and Statistical Manual of Mental Disorders* [DSM] definition), given classical dynamic-psychoanalytic approaches' unsatisfactory response. Over time, it became clear that impairment of the ability to mentalize entails various emotional disturbances and other symptoms, and this method became widely used.

MBT was developed by British psychoanalysts Peter Fonagy, Anthony Bateman, and Mary Target (Bateman & Fonagy, 2004a, 2004b; Bateman & Fonagy, 2006). It is an approach that links classical (Winnicott) and contemporary psychoanalytic (relational) theories, on the one hand, with research approaches in the field of developmental (Bowlby's attachment theory) and cognitive theory (Baron-Cohen's theory of mind), on the other. It is based on the cognitive-developmental theory of mind and assumes that we intuitively create preconceptions and explanations of behavior from infancy. This mentalization includes an ability to think about thoughts, beliefs, emotions, and wishes – our own and those of others – and understand that these internal events variously affect our own, as well as others' behavior. A rigid and non-mentalizing position will be reflected in monolithic, one-track thinking, while a mentalizing attitude is manifested in the ability to raise several alternative possibilities (Diamant, 2008).

The approach also refers to Winnicott when it argues that mentalizing ability depends on how the caregiver reflects the infant's experience to it. The caregiver shows the infant that what the latter sees reflects its own feelings rather than those of the career herself. This reflection allows the infant to understand that what it feels is not the same as others.

Another point of reference for the theory of mind is Bowlby's developmental theory. It claims that the most significant factor in the development of mentalization is secure attachment relations. Having experienced a secure basis, the infant can gain confidence to explore the world – not only around it but also the inner world, of self and others alike.

Though this approach is considered to be psychoanalytic, it implements interventions that are more reminiscent of cognitive-behavioral methods. Fonagy and Bateman argue that in the case of borderline personality disorder, therapy must focus on enhancing the ability to mentalize rather than encouraging insight through interpretations of the transference. To achieve healthy mentalization, the therapist enables the patient to understand things differently and from a number of viewpoints. Being given impulsive reactions to their emotions, borderline patients are asked to suspend their reactions and thoughts. They are required to process their emotions more appropriately and cultivate a better understanding of other people's perspectives.

So classical psychoanalytic practices are significantly different from MBT. In this case, too, the dialectical process can explain a great deal about how they have come to interrelate, with MBT continuing to identify itself as a psychoanalytic approach, acknowledging its roots in the tradition (especially in object relations theory). Fonagy and Bateman, in fact, claim that every therapeutic act includes elements of mentalization so that MBT is not all that innovative. Psychoanalysis, they argue, has always been about recovering the ability to mentalize. It allows the patient to think or reflect on their actions and take an interest in and observe their own and others' consciousness in the secure attachment of the therapeutic relationship. According to Allen (2006), mentalizing is developing awareness of the connections between triggering events in current attachment relationships and previous traumatic experiences. Also cultivating awareness of the impact of one's behavior on attachment figures, an idea originated in Freud's ideas: "Remembering, repeating, and working-through" (Freud, 1914–1958). Allen also indicates that the concept of psychological mindedness is linked to that of insight. Mentalizing highlights the process by focusing on mental activity while insight emphasizes the content.

Through its emphasis on cognition and thought processes and thinking about thinking formerly seen as extraneous to psychoanalysis, the current presence of cognition in the psychoanalytic mainstream no longer takes its cognitive-behavioral form or its older roots. Now cognition flourishes as an integral component of psychoanalysis, fitting in with its developmental theory, its psychopathology, and therapeutic practice. Thus, for instance, we can see how transference relations have been transforming a classic response to the interpretation of unconscious conflict: a systematic effort is now underway to develop the patient's ability to look at her- or himself and others and to build an intelligent look at interpersonal experiential contexts that will help them regulate themselves emotionally. Unlike classical psychoanalysis, this approach abandons the relatively avoidant therapeutic position and the use of in-depth interpretations that involve historical aspects. This model, instead, assumes a more structured and active therapeutic position. It ignores unconscious contents for the benefit of conscious or near-conscious ones. Focusing exclusively on the patient's present mental condition (thoughts, emotions, wishes, desires), the therapist aims to establish the foundations of mental states.

We can put this as follows in Hegelian dialectical terms: While development grounds itself as an outcome of the classical tradition (by viewing pathology as an injury sustained in early attachment relations and in internalized object relations – in theory – and the transference, in practice), the big changes the tradition has undergone are conspicuous: self parts originally negated as being foreign – mainly cognition (in addition to focusing on the present, and therapists' active intervention, in clinical practice) – have been received back in nonidentical form (i.e., mentalization). Even though in this move, the cognitive component of psychoanalysis has been restored through sublation, linking between cognition and behavior – a development ostensibly directly deriving from cognitive-behavioral approaches – the mainstream psychoanalytic approach explicitly rejects behaviorist interventions and safeguards its own focus on the patient's consciousness rather than their behavior (in other words, the intrapsychic aspect). Specific components have to keep being rejected as extraneous to enable distinct, though not fully independent, identity formation. This preserves a dialectic tension in the identity of the approach and its body of knowledge.

To conclude, investigation and observation, in a dialectic development, starts off at a certain point; this process of self-examination exposes inner contradiction, and this contradiction leads to another, new position. This new position negates the previous one, issues from it, and advances from it. Thus, in this process of sublation, the earlier condition, its negation, as well as the new condition are all included. In this dialectic, the two sides of the dialectical tension do not merely coexist; they actually entail one another: necessarily and methodically. That is to say, one does not exist and has no value in the absence of the other (Shalgi, 2009).

It could be said that when assimilating alien concepts or constructs and attributing a new status to them, the risk is to multiply theoretical constructs which refer to the same piece of reality or phenomenon. Katzko (2002) calls this shortcoming "The Uniqueness Assumption" (263):

> The uniqueness assumption typologies an observational level of discourse to reflect theoretical distinctions… Another experimenter, manipulating a different set of variables and using the uniqueness assumption to explain the data will by definition create a theory different from the first. The seed is now sown for a proliferation of mutually exclusive theoretical terminologies.
>
> (p. 265)

This is all truer to grand theories in psychotherapies who rarely use objective, independent evidence. Instead, data are part of the theory and not different from the theory. Theories that endorse previously negated elements implicitly support the uniqueness assumption by not addressing other possible influences if they are not part of their theoretical model. We cannot fully address this problem here, but we would like to mention that Katzko expects psychological research to follow the rules of strict science. This expectation is, of course, highly controversial in our field and a topic of endless debates. Besides having an empirical scientific side, psychology theory (especially psychotherapy) also offers a net of meanings, an ethic, a way to live in the world (Makari, 2000). This will seem from a scientific perspective to be unsystematic but take meaning through historical analysis.

The Scientific Status of Psychoanalysis and Shifts in Epistemological Positioning

One of the main controversies within psychoanalysis is its scientific status. Here we would like to address the relationship between this controversy and dialectics briefly.

We have described the dialectics between psychoanalysis and nonanalytic theories, but there is also another important dialectic in the field of the epistemology of psychoanalysis. The controversy over the scientific status of psychoanalysis cannot be fully addressed here, but it is important to note some important shifts in epistemological positioning that have occurred and the relation of this controversy to dialectics.

Hegel's dialectics epistemology is not just a theory of general knowledge but also a theory of scientific knowledge. As mentioned before, for Hegel a knowledge entity develops as a subject-like structure and comes into being in the same manner as self-consciousness. For Hegel, science is the totality of its components. Developments in science constitute the developmental stages, each one including those that came before it.

Up until the 1970s, most psychoanalysts followed Freud's scientific worldview and were committed to the idea that psychoanalysis is a science, and that meant devising a mechanistic theory to explain normal and abnormal thought (Basch, 1993). In the last decades, there was a radical shift, and many scholars suggested modern hermeneutics and postmodernism as better epistemologies. Others seek a more intermediate position between science and hermeneutics (Makari, 2000; Negri et al., 2019). Fusella (2014) argues that psychoanalysis has situated itself among the other disciplines as a hybrid science, not quite a pure hermeneutic, on the one hand, and not quite a pure science, on the other.

The change in epistemological positioning in the scientific discourse can also be seen in the disagreements about empirical evidence and the evaluation of psychoanalysis (e.g., Hoffman [2009] and Safran [2012], response). Hoffman thinks that systematic empirical research on psychotherapy process and outcome is less relevant for psychoanalysis than the traditional case studies. In contrast, Safran (2012) describes a middle ground approach to science which recognizes that "science has an irreducibly social, hermeneutic, and political character, and that data are only one element in an ongoing conversation between members of a scientific community" (p. 710). While positivism argues for only one path to truth, hermeneutics believes that there is more than one truth. Its interest is in emergent processes and moral commitments to self-reflection and critical thought (Cushman, 2013).

It seems that relational theory has shifted away from realist aspirations or impersonal objectivity to the creative power of human imagination as regards subjectivity, intersubjectivity, and truth (Elliott & Spezzano, 1996). Moreover, some postmodern discourses have sought to attack the scientific worldview and undermine scientific truths in order to undermine science (Kuntz, 2012). However, it is to the credit of the postmodern thinkers in relational psychoanalysis that they have insisted on rejecting radical antiscientist postmodernism as an appropriate epistemology for psychoanalysis. In a manner often seen in dialectical development, the relational tradition has, in fact, had a positive impact on certain aspects of psychoanalysis. Postmodern approaches such as the relational approach do not necessarily lead to rejecting data, which are still a central source of intersubjective knowledge. Instead, the very acknowledgment that data necessarily requires interpretation entails a renewed centrality of data themselves. Also, postmodern theories do not necessarily mean that realism is false; the acknowledgment that objectivity is always intersubjectivity doesn't necessarily clash with a contemporary view of science. Osbeck (2019), for example, offers a holistic picture of the scientific project that acknowledges the role of imagination, perspective-taking, and values alongside observation and reason. For her, foregrounding "the personal" also emphasizes continuity across arts and sciences, the interfaces of which contain the full range of resources for innovative thinking.

We believe that such postmodern approaches are dialectical by their nature in incorporating antagonists and contradictions. Here too, dialectics appears to be relevant. For example, classical psychoanalysts who tend to perceive psychoanalysis as a scientific discipline and to endorse realism and the correspondence theory of truth vehemently oppose scientific evidence of all sorts, particularly when it derives from nonanalytic theories (as in Blass and Carmeli [2007] criticism of neuropsychoanalysis, and Green [2000] criticism against infant research). At the same time, the relational theoreticians were the first to endorse psychoanalytically informed infant research based on systematic observations on parent-infant interaction outside psychoanalysis. Benjamin (2013) writes:

.... infancy research electrified me. What awesome possibilities it seemed to open up, is what I felt when I first encountered the work of Stern (1974a, b) and Beebe (Beebe & Stern, 1977) in 1978. Face-to-face play was the primary illustration of how mutual recognition is possible so early! ...As it now seemed that all roads were leading to recognition and intersubjectivity, somehow I had to get them all on the same map.

(p. 4)

Here again, objective science was negated but then returned in a different form as representing intersubjectivity, a term that infant researchers like Stern (1974a) use for lack of a better word. Paradoxically, infant research is incorporated in a postmodern approach not only for its systematic and evidence-based methods but for its detailed description of recognition and intersubjectivity. Likewise, classical psychoanalysts show indifference to nonanalytic theories but only after the psychoanalytic theories are well founded. Steiner (2000) notes that

there is no doubt that extra-analytical observations played a certain role in confirming and refining, at times, Freud's and the first child analysts' observations and hypotheses concerning the chronology of the development of the internal life of the baby and the child.

(p. 10)

Steiner shows that in the phase of imagining a new infant, Winnicott, Klein, Lacan, and others used nonanalytic theories to validate their new theories of development.

Future Application

Mainstream psychoanalysis has, as said, invested significant resources to defend its boundaries from external influences. This jealous self-protection requires an investment in keeping the self and others apart. Any attempt at development within the discipline requires proof that new ideas don't smuggle in foreign elements – which will meet rejection. However, we have seen that from a dialectical perspective, any development, any movement ahead, necessarily involves such foreign elements. This is a foreignness that should not be considered only extraneous to psychoanalysis.

In this chapter, we offer a new perspective on interdisciplinarity in the psycho-analytic clinic. Rather than either isolationism or an externally imposed alienated unity in the face of the other, we have sought to reflect on psychoanalysis's encounter with other theories in terms of a dialectical movement within psychoanalysis itself. Here the other, nonanalytical approach is seen to constitute an integral moment in the development of psychoanalytic knowledge.

Distinction and emphasizing salient differences between the schools in the field of psychotherapy is made in purpose to sustain professional-cultural identity. Psychoanalysis needs to hold convictions about what it believes and what it rejects for a stable and robust identity. As a result, mental barriers are formed which keep out the threat and keep the subject at a safe intellectual distance. This phenomenon is not unique to psychoanalysis; Wachtel (2010, 2018) sees the field of psychotherapy as divided between "tribal organizations" entangled in a culture war, something more like an ethnic conflict with its attendant us-vs-them feelings than an intellectual or scientific discussion. Differences are polarized; caricature and stereotype abound; each side is intensely attached to its own way, and self-definition is achieved by diminishing the other. "What lies outside might be not only not noticed but actively rejected since it is associated with a point of view that is derided and disdained as 'other,'" in Wachtel's words (Wachtel, 2010, p. 407). It seems that no school of therapy appears to have a monopoly on dogmatism or therapeutic insensitivity (Shedler, 2010).

Authors writing about fragmentation, disunity, and the crisis of the field have been facing the problem from perspectives ranging from political viewpoints to rhetorical, via theoretical-methodological, historical, educational, and meta-theoretical levels of inquiry and also as a sociocultural phenomenon including organizational processes and traditional communities (Gaj, 2016). Many clinicians have sought to offer a solution to this disunity in the field – at the theoretical level by trans-theoretical approaches (Prochaska & DiClemente, 2019) and at the research level of evaluation findings by developing near-optimal systematic statistical prediction rules that should be used in preference to intuition (Dawes, 2005). Hegel's dialectics may offer another solution that does not seek unity in conformity of method or theory.

We believe that actively encouraging the position of reflection and self-skepticism and openness to and acknowledging the other, by knowing the dialectic, is of great importance:

Through mutual recognition, each discipline moves closer to appreciating the value of the other, and this process is what advances knowledge. Like spirit, which seeks recognition from the other so that it may recover its lost alienated desire, mutual recognition provides mutual validation and acceptance, which opens up further communication and dialogue.

(Mills, 2012, p. 192)

Hegel's dialectical development of the subject or of subject-like structures like psychoanalysis is a description of how things evolve naturally as we constitute ourselves and our knowledge. It is true that according to the dialectics, only in the affirmation of identity, difference, and then subsequently sublation can the process of knowledge proceed. At the same time, developments in psychotherapy in general and in psychoanalysis, in particular, occur in different ways through exposure to the other (e.g., Peri Herzovich & Govrin, 2021). According to this, we believe that when psychoanalysis can identify itself by finding itself in its other and by finding the other within itself – which is tantamount to acknowledging its own self-difference or alienation – it will have an ability to expose itself to other theories to conduct a respectful and stimulating interaction. This would in fact be its way of maintaining its separate identity, exactly through acknowledging extra-analytical bodies of knowledge and its own position vis-à-vis them.

Psychoanalysis will reap multiple benefits from its interest in these different theories. It will get to know itself better and allow for self-criticism, questions, and doubt, and it will be open to consider its own shortcomings. This will help it avoid paralysis, dwindling creativity, and growing irrelevant and outdated.

In an era marked by frequent change, psychoanalysis cannot afford to remain stuck. To stay in contact with developments and remain relevant, it needs to foster its ability to find sustenance outside itself – as long as that sustenance does not threaten its continued existence. We suggest that rather than directing its efforts to put up walls and ignoring other, non-psychoanalytic approaches, psychoanalysis should look for its commonalities with them – first, as it looks inward and then to confidently open itself to such encounters and even encourage them. According to the dialectical process, growth is enabled by the other but confirms the self insofar as it must be able to recognize the other.

To conclude, while psychoanalysis defines itself by reference to what it is not, its development necessitates an ability to recognize that what is extraneous to itself is also part of itself. When it acknowledges its other, psychoanalysis recognizes its own otherness or its multiple nature. This forms simultaneously, and dialectically, a recognition of its own unity.

References

Allen, J. G. (2006). Mentalizing in practice. In J. G. Allen, & P. Fonagy, (Eds.), *The handbook of mentalization-based treatment* (pp. 3–30). Chichester; West Sussex: John Wiley & Sons Ltd. http://doi.org/10.1002/9780470712986.ch1

Basch, M. F. (1993). Comments on the scientific status of psychoanalysis. *The Journal of Psychotherapy Practice and Research, 2*, 185–190.

Bateman, A. W., & Fonagy, P. (2004a). Mentalization-based treatment of BPD. *The Journal of Personality Disorders, 18*, 36–51. http://doi.org/10.1521/pedi.18.1.36.32772

Bateman, A. W., & Fonagy, P. (2004b). *Psychotherapy for borderline personality disorder: Mentalization-based treatment.* New York: Oxford University Press. http://doi.org/10.1093/med:psych/9780198527664.001.0001

Bateman, A. W., & Fonagy, P. (2006). *Mentalization-Based Treatment for Borderline Personality Disorder: A Practical Guide*. New York: Oxford University Press. http://doi.org/10.1093/med/9780198570905.001.0001

Beebe, B., & Stern, D. (1977). Engagement-disengagement and early object experiences. In N. Freedman & S. Grand (Eds.), *Communicative structures and psychic structures* (pp. 35–55). New York: Plenum.

Benjamin, J. (2013). The bonds of love: Looking backward. *Studies in Gender and Sexuality, 14*, 1–15. http://doi.org/10.1080/15240657.2013.756769

Berman, E. (2010). On 'affirming "that's not psychoanalysis!." *The International Journal of Psychoanalysis, 91*, 1281–1282. http://doi.org/10.1111/j.1745–8315.2010.00349.x

Blass, R. B. (2010). Affirming "that's not psychoanalysis!" On the value of the politically incorrect act of attempting to define the limits of our field. *The International Journal of Psychoanalysis, 91*, 81–99. http://doi.org/10.1111/j.1745–8315.2009.00211.x

Blass, R. B., & Carmeli, Z. (2007). The case against neuropsychoanalysis. *The International Journal of Psychoanalysis, 88*, 19–40. http://doi.org/10.1516/6NCA-A4MA-MFQ7-0JTJ

Bornstein, R. F. (2001). The impending death of psychoanalysis. *Psychoanalytic psychology, 18*, 3–20. http://doi.org/10.1037/0736–9735.18.1.2

Boswell, J. F., Sharpless, B. A., Greenberg, L. S., Heatherington, L., Huppert, J. D., Barber, J. P., et al. (2010). Schools of psychotherapy and the beginnings of a scientific approach. In D. H. Barlow (Ed.), *The oxford handbook of clinical psychology* (pp. 98–127). Oxford: Oxford University Press. http://doi.org/10.1093/oxfordhb/9780195366884.013.0006

Brenner, C. (1968). Psychanalysais and science. *The Journal of the American Psychoanalytic Association, 16*, 675–696. http://doi.org/10.1177/000306516801600401

Butterfield, H. (1997 [1957]). *The origins of modern science (Vol. 90507)*. New York: Simon and Schuster Inc.

Carr, E., & Cortina, M. (2011). Heinz Kohut and John Bowlby: The men and their ideas. *Psychoanalytic Inquiry, 31*, 42–57. http://doi.org/10.1080/07351690.2010.512847

Castiglioni, M., & Corradini, A. (2011). *Modelli Epistemologici in Psicologia, [Epistemological models in psychology]* (2nd Ed.). Roma: Carocci.

Cherry, S., Meyer, J., Mann, G., & Meersand, P. (2020). Professional and personal development after psychoanalytic training: Interviews with early career analysts. *The Journal of the American Psychoanalytic Association, 68*, 217–239. http://doi.org/10.1177/0003065120921563

Cohen, I. B. (1985). *Revolution in science*. Cambridge, MA: The Belknap Press of the Harvard University Press.

Cohen, R. S., & Wartofsky, M. W. (Eds.). (1984). *Hegel and the sciences* (Vol. 64). Dordrecht: Springer. http://doi.org/10.1007/978–94–009–6233-0

Cushman, P. (2013). Because the rock will not read the article: A discussion of Jeremy D. Safran's critique of Irwin Z. Hoffman's "doublethinking our way to scientific legitimacy." *Psychoanalytic Dialogues, 23*, 211–224. http://doi.org/10.1080/10481885.2013.772478

Davanloo, H. (1978). *Basic principles and techniques in short-term dynamic psychotherapy*. New York: Spectrum.

Davanloo, H. (1980). *Short-term dynamic psychotherapy*. New York: Jason Aronson.

Dawes, R. M. (2005). The ethical implications of Paul Meehl's work on comparing clinical versus actuarial prediction methods. *Journal of Clinical Psychology, 61*, 1245–1255. http://doi.org/10.1002/jclp.20180

Diamant, I. (2008). *In a Nutshell: The practice of mentalizing based treatment and the therapeutic practice of borderline personality disorder*. Available online at: https://www.hebpsy.net/articles.asp?id=1875 (accessed April, 11, 2021).

Donovan, J. M. (1987). Brief dynamic psychotherapy: Toward a more comprehensive model. *Psychiatry* 50, 167–183.

Elliott, A., & Spezzano, C. (1996). Psychoanalysis at its limits: Navigating the postmodern turn. *Psychoanal. Q.* 65, 52–83. http://doi.org/10.1080/21674086.1996.11927483

Erickson, M. H. (1954). Special techniques of brief hypnotherapy. *International Journal of Clinical and Experimental Hypnosis, 2,* 109–129. http://doi.org/10.1080/00207145408409943

Freud, S. (1905). Jokes and their relation to the unconscious. In J. Strachey (Ed.), *The standard edition of the complete psychological works of Sigmund Freud* (Vol. 8, pp. 1–247). London: Hogarth Press.

Freud, S. (1912). Recommendations to physicians practicing psychoanalysis. In J. Strachey (Ed.), *The standard edition of the complete psychological works of Sigmund Freud* (Vol. 12, pp. 109–120). London: Hogarth Press.

Freud, S. (1914–1958). Remembering, repeating, and working-through. In J. Strachey (Ed.), *The standard edition of the complete psychological works of Sigmund Freud* (Vol. 12, pp. 147–156). London: Hogarth Press.

Freud, S. (1915). Observations on transference-love (further recommendations on the technique of psychoanalysis III). In J. Strachey (Ed.), *The standard edition of the complete psychological works of Sigmund Freud* (Vol. 12, pp. 157–171). London: Hogarth Press.

Freud, S. (1919). The *"Uncanny"*. *The standard edition of the complete psychological works of Sigmund Freud, Volume XVII (1917–1919): An infantile neurosis and other works* (pp. 217–256). London: Hogarth Press.

Freud, S. (1921). Group psychology and the analysis of the ego. In J. Strachey (Ed.), *The standard edition of the complete psychological works of Sigmund Freud* (Vol. 18, pp. 65–144). London: Hogarth Press.

Freud, S., & Breuer, J. (1955/1895). Studies in hysteria. In J. Strachey (Ed.), *The standard edition of the complete psychological works of Sigmund Freud* (Vol. 2). London: Hogarth Press.

Fritsch, R. C., & Winer, R. (2020). Combined training of candidates, scholars, and psychotherapists: A model of psychoanalytic education for the twenty-first century. *Journal of the American Psychoanalytic Association, 68,* 175–200. http://doi.org/10.1177/0003065120922846

Fusella, P. (2014). Hermeneutics versus science in psychoanalysis: A resolution to the controversy over the scientific status of psychoanalysis. *Psychoanalytic Review, 101,* 871–894. http://doi.org/10.1521/prev.2014.101.6.871

Gaj, N. (2016). *Unity and fragmentation in psychology: The philosophical and methodological roots of the discipline.* London: Routledge. http://doi.org/10.4324/9781315652573

Govrin, A. (2004). *Between abstinence and seduction.* Tel Aviv: Kinneret, Zmora-Bitan, Dvir.

Govrin, A. (2015). *Conservative and radical perspectives on psychoanalytic knowledge: The fascinated and the disenchanted.* London: Routledge. http://doi.org/10.4324/9781315719153

Govrin, A. (2016). Blurring the threat of "otherness": Integration by conversion in psychoanalysis and CBT. *Journal of Psychotherapy Integration, 26,* 78–90. http://doi.org/10.1037/a0039637

Green, A. (2000). Science and science fiction in infant research. In J. Sandler, A. M. Sandler, & R. Davies (Eds.), *Clinical and observational psychoanalytic research: Roots of a controversy* (pp. 41–72). Madison, CT: International Universities Press. http://doi.org/10.4324/9780429472923-5

Gurman, A. S., & Kniskern, D. P. (1981–1991). *Handbook of family therapy* (Vols. I and II). New York: Brunner/Mazel.

Gustafson, J. P. (1984). An integration of brief dynamic psychotherapy. *American Journal of Psychiatry, 141*, 935–944. http://doi.org/10.1176/ajp.141.8.935

Haley, J. (1963). *Strategies of psychotherapy.* New York: Grune and Stratton. http://doi.org/10.1037/14324-000

Hegel, G. W. F. (1892a). *Lectures on history and philosophy* (Vol. 3). London: Routledge and Kegan Paul.

Hegel, G. W. F. (1892b). *The logic of Hegel (From Encyclopaedia)* (2nd ed.). Oxford: Oxford University Press.

Hegel, G. W. F. (1956/1837). *The philosophy of history.* New York: Dover.

Hegel, G. W. F. (1969/1812). *The science of logic.* London: George Allen and Unwin.

Hegel, G. W. F. (2018/1807). *The phenomenology of spirit.* Oxford: Oxford University Press.

Hoffman, I. Z. (2009). Doublethinking our way to "scientific" legitimacy: The desiccation of human experience. *Journal of the American Psychoanalytic Association, 57*, 1043–1069. http://doi.org/10.1177/0003065109343925

Jones, E. (1955). *The life and work of Sigmund Freud, Vol. 2: Years of maturity 1901–1919.* London: Hogarth Press.

Kahn, E., & Rachman, A. W. (2000). Carl Rogers and Heinz Kohut: A historical perspective. *Psychoanalytic Psychology, 17*, 294–312. http://doi.org/10.1037/0736–9735.17.2.294

Katzko, M. W. (2002). The rhetoric of psychological research and the problem of unification in psychology. *American Psychology, 57*, 262–270. http://doi.org/10.1037/0003–066X.57.4.262

Kohut, H. (1959). Introspection, empathy, and psychoanalysis: An examination of the relationship between mode of observation and theory. *Journal of the American Psychoanalytic Association, 7*, 459–483. http://doi.org/10.1177/000306515900700304

Kohut, H. (1971). *The analysis of the self.* New York: International Universities Press.

Kohut, H. (1975). The psychoanalyst in the community of scholars. *Annual of Psychoanalysis, 3*, 341–370.

Kohut, H. (1977). *The restoration of the self.* New York: International Universities Press.

Kohut, H. (1978). *The search for the self, Vol. 1 and 2.* New York: International Universities Press.

Kohut, H. (1984). *How does analysis cure?* Chicago, IL: The University of Chicago Press. http://doi.org/10.7208/chicago/9780226006147.001.0001

Kristeva, J. (1991/1988). *Strangers to ourselves.* New York: Columbia University Press.

Kuntz, M. (2012). The postmodern assault on science. *Scientific Societies, 13*, 885–889. http://doi.org/10.1038/embor.2012.130

Lemma, A., Target, M., & Fonagy, P. (2010). The development of a brief psychodynamic protocol for depression: Dynamic interpersonal therapy (DIT). *Psychoanalytic Psychotherapy, 24*, 329–346. http://doi.org/10.1080/02668734.2010.513547

Levkovich, R. E. (2011). *Reviewed works: The tragedy in ethical life: Hegel's philosophy and the spirit of modernity by Pini Ifergan* (pp. 383–393). Iyyun: The Jerusalem Philosophical Quarterly.

Luborsky, L. (1984). *Principles of psychoanalytic psychotherapy. A manual for supportive-expressive psychotherapy.* New York: Basic Books.

Makari, G. J. (2000). Change in psychoanalysis: Science, practice, and the sociology of knowledge. In P. Fonagy, R. Michels, & J. Sandler (Eds.), *Changing ideas in a changing world: The revolution in psychoanalysis: Essays in honour of Arnold Cooper* (pp. 255–262). London: Karnac Books.

Malan, D. H. (1963). *A study of brief psychotherapy.* Oxford: Charles C Thomas.

Malan, D. H. (1976). *Toward the validation of dynamic psychotherapy: A replication.* Oxford: Plenum. http://doi.org/10.1007/978-1-4615-8753-8

Malcolm, J. (1982). *Psychoanalysis: The impossible profession.* New York: Knopf Doubleday Publishing Group; Vintage Books.

Mann, J. (1973). *Time-limited psychotherapy.* Cambridge, MA: Harvard University Press.

Mann, J., & Goldman, R. (1982). *A casebook in time-limited psychotherapy.* New York: McGraw-Hill.

Menaker, E. (1978). Kohut's restoration of the self: A symposium. *Psychoanalytic Review, 65,* 620–622.

Migone, P. (2011). On: The definition of psychoanalysis. *International Journal of Psychoanalysis, 92,* 1315–1317. http://doi.org/10.1111/j.1745–8315.2011.00431.x

Milchman, A., & Rosenberg, A. (2011). A Foucauldian analysis of psychoanalysis: A discipline that disciplines. Academy for the Psychoanalytic Arts. https://academyanalyticarts. org/milchman-foucauldian-analysis (Accessed May 31, 2021).

Mills, J. (2012). *The unconscious Abyss: Hegel's anticipation of psychoanalysis.* Albany: SUNY Press.

Miltone, J. (2001). Psychoanalysis and cognitive behavior therapy – rival paradigms or common ground? *International Journal of Psychoanalysis, 82,* 431–446. http://doi.org/10.1516/ DVLN-RK5E-C1YV-ME4V

Moses, I. (1988). The misuse of empathy in psychoanalysis. *Contemporary Psychoanalysis, 24,* 577–594. http://doi.org/10.1080/00107530.1988.10746265

Negri, A., Andreoli, G., Belotti, L., Barazzetti, A., & Martin, E. H. (2019). Psychotherapy trainees' epistemological assumptions influencing research-practice integration. *Research in Psychotherapy, 22,* 344–358. http://doi.org/10.4081/ripppo.2019.397

Osbeck, L. (2019). *Values in psychological science: Re-imagining epistemic priorities at a new Frontier.* Cambridge: Cambridge University Press.

Peri Herzovich, Y., & Govrin, A. (2021). Psychoanalysis and CBT: From rivalry to hospitality in psychotherapy integration. *British Journal of Psychotherapy, 37,* 244–262. http:// doi.org/10.1111/bjp.12625

Prochaska, J. O., & DiClemente, C. C. (2019). The transtheoretical approach. In J. C. Norcross, & M. R. Goldfried (Eds.), *Handbook of psychotherapy integration* (pp. 161–183). New York: Oxford University Press. http://doi.org/10.1093/med-psych/9780190690465.003.0008

Reik, T. (1960). *The haunting melody: Psychoanalytic experiences in life and music.* Oxford: Grove.

Rogers, C. R. (1942). *Counseling and psychotherapy: Newer concepts in practice.* Oxford: Houghton Mifflin.

Safran, J. D. (2012). Doublethinking or dialectical thinking: A critical appreciation of Hoffman's "doublethinking" critique. *Psychoanalytic Dialogues, 22,* 710–720. http://doi.org/ 10.1080/10481885.2012.733655

Safran, J. D., & Messer, S. B. (1997). Psychotherapy integration: A postmodern critique. *Clinical Psychology, 4,* 140–152. http://doi.org/10.1111/j.1468–2850.1997.tb00106.x

Sampson, E. E. (1993). *Celebrating the other: A dialogic account of human nature.* Boulder, CO: Westview Press.

Schwartz, L. (1978). The restoration of the self: By Heinz Kohut, M. D. *Psychoanalytic Quarterly,* 47, 436–443.

Shahar, G. (2011). Israeli clinical psychology – where to? *Conversations Israel Journal of Psychotherapy, 26,* 1–7.

Shalgi, B. (2009). Three dimensions of the human existence: The contribution of Hegel's philosophy to intersubjective psychoanalysis. *Conversations Israel Journal of Psychotherapy, 24,* 25–39.

Shedler, J. (2010). The efficacy of psychodynamic psychotherapy. *American Psychologist, 65,* 98–109. http://doi.org/10.1037/a0018378

Shedler, J. (2015). Where is the evidence for "evidence based" psychotherapy? *Journal of Psychology Therapy Primary Care, 4,* 47–59.

Sifneos, P. E. (1972). *Short term psychotherapy and emotional crisis.* Boston, MA: Harvard University Press.

Sifneos, P. E. (1979). *Short-term dynamic psychotherapy: Evaluation and technique.* New York: Plenum. http://doi.org/10.1007/978-1-4684-3530-6

Sorenson, R. L. (2000). Psychoanalytic institutes as religious denominations: Fundamentalism, progeny, and ongoing reformation. *Psychoanalytic Dialogues, 10,* 847–874. http://doi.org/10.1080/10481881009348587

Stein, M. H. (1979). *The restoration of the self: By Heinz Kohut.* New York: International Universities Press.

Steiner, R. (1991). Background to the scientific controversies. In P. King & R. Steiner (Eds.), *New Library of Psychoanalysis, No.* 11. *The Freud-Klein Controversies 1941–45* (pp. 227–263). London: Routledge.

Steiner, R. (2000). Introduction. In J. Sandler, A. Sandler, & R. Davies (Eds.), *Clinical and observational psychoanalytic research: Roots of a controversy* (pp. 1–20). Madison, CT: International Universities Press.

Stern, D. N. (1974a). Mother and infant at play: The dyadic interaction involving facial, vocal, and gaze behaviors. In M. Lewis & L. A. Rosenblum (Eds.), *The effect of the infant on its caregiver* (pp. 187–213). Oxford: Wiley-Interscience.

Stern, D. N. (1974b). The goal and structure of mother-infant play. *Journal of the American Academy of Child & Adolescent Psychiatry, 13,* 402–421.

Strupp, H. H., & Binder, J. L. (1984). *Psychotherapy in a new key: A guide to time limited psychotherapy.* New York: Basic Books.

Thagard, P. (1982). Hegel, science, and set theory. *Erkenntnis, 18,* 397–410. http://doi.org/10.1007/BF00205279

Tobin, S. A. (1991). A comparison of psychoanalytic self psychology and Carl Rogers's person-centered therapy. *Journal of Humanistic Psychology, 31,* 9–33. http://doi.org/10.1177/0022167891311002

Wachtel, P. L. (2010). Psychotherapy integration and integrative psychotherapy: Process or product? *Journal of Psychotherapy Integration, 20,* 406–416. http://doi.org/10.1037/a0022032

Wachtel, P. L. (2018). Pathways to progress for integrative psychotherapy: Perspectives on practice and research. *Journal of Psychotherapy Integration, 28,* 202–212. http://doi.org/10.1037/int0000089

Westen, D., Novotny, C. M., & Thompson-Brenner, H. (2004). The empirical status of empirically supported psychotherapies: Assumptions, findings, and reporting in controlled clinical trials. *Psychol. Bull.* 130, 631–663. http://doi.org/10.1037/0033-2909.130.4.631

Yovel, Y. (1975). Hegel on reason, actuality and philosophical discourse. *Iyyun: The Jerusalem Philosophical Quarterly, 26*(1–3), 59–115.

Yovel, Y. (2001). Introduction. In G. W. F. Hegel (ed.), *Preface to phenomenology of spirit* (pp. 13–47). Jerusalem: Magnes.

Chapter 5

Fusion of Horizons in Psychotherapy Integration

A Dialogue Between Psychoanalysis and Cognitive-Behavioral Therapy

Yael Peri Herzovich

This final chapter explores the essence of psychotherapy integration as a dialogue between different approaches, focusing on psychoanalysis and cognitive-behavioral therapy (CBT) as exemplars of rival schools in the field. Among the significant obstacles to dialogue are practitioners' fear of losing their distinct professional identities and the substantial gaps between different therapeutic cultures. This raises a crucial question: How can dialogue between different psychotherapeutic schools be facilitated in a way that acknowledges and preserves, rather than diminishes, their cultural and theoretical differences? Drawing on Gadamer's hermeneutics, we propose that these very differences, initially perceived as obstacles, may hold the key to meaningful dialogue. According to Gadamer, dialogue occurs between the horizons of different traditions, where tradition encompasses the sum of prejudices through which people relate to the world – including beliefs, information, concepts, perceptions, and internalized values. The horizon, in Gadamer's view, represents the range of vision that includes everything perceived from a particular vantage point. Understanding the other in dialogue is shaped precisely by these prejudices derived from one's cultural tradition. For Gadamer, understanding is a process of "fusion of horizons." This fusion does not imply agreement; rather, it suggests that the prejudices inherent in one tradition can facilitate understanding of an entirely different tradition, leading to deeper and broader self-understanding through engagement with the other's perspective. We argue that through engagement with other psychotherapeutic schools, each therapeutic tradition can gain new insights about itself and expand its horizons. This perspective allows for growth and development while maintaining the distinctiveness of each tradition. Through such dialogue, psychotherapeutic schools can preserve their uniqueness and minimize threats to professional-cultural identity while fostering openness, receptivity, and mutual development. Although Gadamer does not advocate a methodical approach, his ideas provide a framework for understanding the conditions necessary for productive dialogue between different psychotherapeutic schools.

DOI: 10.4324/9781003608103-6

Psychotherapy Integration: The Call for Dialogue

Wachtel, P.L.: "When you have two clinicians up here and they're savvy toward each other, it's a bit rough. What I am hoping for and still am is, first of all, dialogue. I think one of the things that struck me was that there was very little dialogue among theoretical orientations. I think SEPI has been very successful, but there's still a lot of separate worlds that don't hear each other, that don't know about each other, that don't take each other seriously, and most of all don't learn from each other."

(Wachtel & Goldfried, 2005, p. 499)

The quest for dialogue between psychotherapeutic approaches emerged in the 1930s, when pioneers in the field began advocating for integration across different schools of thought. This movement gained significant momentum during the 1980s, culminating in the establishment of the Society for the Exploration of Psychotherapy Integration (SEPI) (Goldfried et al., 2019). The primary mission of SEPI was to foster meaningful dialogue and exchange among clinicians and researchers from diverse theoretical orientations. In its early years, SEPI organized numerous conferences and meetings, not to create integrative models, but rather to facilitate genuine dialogue between different perspectives on theory, clinical practice, and research (Goldfried et al., 2005).

While dialogue between approaches remained a central goal of the integration movement, over time its focus shifted increasingly toward developing integrative models. This latter form of integration represents an effort to create comprehensive frameworks for understanding human experience and treating psychological distress. This shift reflected a growing recognition that no single approach could address all therapeutic challenges, that significant overlap existed between approaches, and that integration could enhance therapeutic effectiveness (Ziv-Beiman & Shahar, 2014).

Wachtel (2010) articulates this dual nature of integration:

Psychotherapy integration is a term whose connotations are more closely associated with a *process*, whereas integrative psychotherapy can seem to imply a *product*. That is, integration – or integrating – is an ongoing aim or effort or, put differently, it is a road to a destination, a destination which may not even be known or visible as one proceeds. In contrast, integrative psychotherapy suggests an already achieved integration or, to return to the metaphor of the previous sentence, the destination toward which the road has been leading.

(p.411)

This tension between process and product reflects a fundamental debate within the field. While some practitioners advocate for one direction over the other, many argue that the essence of psychotherapy integration lies in maintaining both aspirations. What unifies various perspectives within the integration movement is the shared recognition that the field is constrained by artificial divisions between theoretical approaches – divisions often maintained through mutual disregard or even hostility (Wachtel, 2010). The founding figures of the integration movement consistently emphasize that the commitment to "Exploration" must be preserved – specifically, the ongoing process of self-examination through dialogue with other schools. They caution that abandoning this goal risks reverting to the very isolationism that integration seeks to overcome (Safran & Messer, 1997; Stricker, 2010; Wachtel, 2010).

Despite the integration movement's aspirations, establishing genuine dialogue between different therapeutic approaches has proven challenging. Miller (1992) suggests that the theoretical prestige of individual schools creates nearly insurmountable barriers to theoretical dialogue. In this environment, rational discourse is often replaced by rhetoric and dismissive attitudes, while loyalty to clearly defined theoretical positions leads to rigid, defensive stances that reinforce existing divisions. Miller observes that practitioners from different orientations often treat those who don't share their theoretical framework as "heretics" rather than colleagues whose perspectives deserve consideration. This attitude frames serious engagement with theoretical differences as not merely wasteful but potentially dangerous, risking "contamination" of what Miller terms the therapist's "pure soul."

Building on this observation, Wachtel (2010, 2018) argues that psychotherapeutic schools function essentially as cultural communities, where practitioners forge their professional identities through identification with their therapeutic tradition. Consequently, encounters between psychotherapeutic schools more closely resemble cultural conflicts than intellectual discussions – a form of tribal warfare marked by sharp "us-vs-them" distinctions. These distinctions serve to reinforce each school's identity, with any external influence perceived as threatening to this identity. This perceived threat to professional-cultural identity often prevents genuine openness to alternative perspectives (Peri Herzovich & Govrin, 2021).

A further obstacle emerges in the work of Safran and Messer (1997), who highlight how concepts from one therapeutic tradition often lose their meaning when transplanted into another theoretical context. Goldfried (2019) extends this analysis, noting that the challenge lies not only in differing theories or techniques but in the distinct theoretical languages of each approach. These different conceptual vocabularies create barriers to mutual understanding and learning.

This analysis reveals that barriers to dialogue between psychotherapeutic approaches stem from two main sources. First, practitioners maintain strong attachments to their professional-cultural identities and feel threatened by potential dilution of these identities. Second, the very nature of distinct therapeutic traditions – each with its own language, value system, and practices – creates inherent challenges to mutual understanding.

In light of these challenges, we pose a critical question: How can meaningful dialogue develop between advocates of different psychotherapeutic schools despite these cultural, traditional, and linguistic barriers? This question is crucial not only for the integration movement but for the broader development of psychotherapy as a field, including its various schools, and specifically psychoanalysis and CBT which we address in this chapter.

Since SEPI's establishment, most integration-oriented professionals have focused on identifying common principles and processes of therapeutic change that transcend theoretical boundaries. Their approach emphasizes similarities between different schools rather than differences (Goldfried, 2019; Wachtel, 2018). We propose a different perspective. If the core challenge lies in the cultural, traditional, and linguistic gaps between schools – gaps zealously maintained to preserve distinct professional identities – then emphasizing similarities might paradoxically increase resistance and impede dialogue. This raises several crucial questions: How can we facilitate a genuine exchange between psychotherapy schools by acknowledging, rather than minimizing, their differences? How can two theoretical frameworks that differ fundamentally – from their understanding of human suffering to their views on therapeutic relationships – engage in meaningful dialogue? How can separate professional communities, each with their own organizations, conferences, and journals, develop authentic interest in learning from each other?

In this chapter, we propose a solution that embraces, rather than attempts to overcome, the differences between psychotherapeutic approaches. Drawing on *Gadamer's hermeneutics (1975)*, we suggest that what appears to be the main obstacle to dialogue – the gaps in culture, tradition, and language – may actually hold the key to meaningful exchange.

According to Gadamer, meaningful dialogue occurs between the horizons of different traditions. Understanding emerges not despite but through the prejudices arising from each participant's cultural tradition. For Gadamer, understanding involves a "fusion of horizons" – not a merging or dissolution of differences but a process where the perspectives inherent in one tradition enable understanding of another. This fusion leads to deeper self-understanding through engagement with the other's viewpoint.

This interdisciplinary framework connects philosophical insights about encountering "the other" with the practical challenges of psychotherapy integration. By applying Gadamer's hermeneutic principles to the field of psychotherapy integration, we aim to illuminate new possibilities for meaningful dialogue between psychotherapeutic approaches. We will examine this through the lens of psychoanalysis and CBT, two approaches that represent one of the most pronounced rivalries in the field.

In the following sections, we will present Gadamer's core theoretical principles, demonstrate how psychoanalysis has already incorporated aspects of his thinking, and illustrate how these principles can advance dialogue in psychotherapy integration.

Gadamer's Dialogue

In the second half of the twentieth century, Hans-Georg Gadamer developed his unique hermeneutic approach, detailed in his book *Truth and Method* (1975). Gadamer embraced Heidegger's (1962) view of hermeneutic activity as a central component of human existence, rather than merely a means of gaining knowledge about the world. In essence, to live as a human being is to derive meaning in every moment.

Following this perspective, Gadamer viewed understanding not as a special spiritual act but as the fundamental mode of human existence. In his essay, "The Universality of the Hermeneutical Problem" (1966), Gadamer argued that "Language is the fundamental mode of operation of our being-in-the-world and the all-embracing form of the constitution of the world" (p. 3). Consequently, he proposed a hermeneutics that seeks not only to extract meaning from texts but to observe the process of meaning-making that occurs in every moment of human life through the medium of language.

In *Truth and Method* (1975), Gadamer proposed viewing the hermeneutic relationship as a "dialogue" with the text, conceptualizing the interaction between an interpreter and a text as a relationship between two subjects. This perspective reveals the universal nature of human understanding, where the dialogical relationship between self and other constitutes understanding, whether the other is a text or a subject. Gadamer emphasized that understanding emerges in the encounter between interpreter and text, or between "I" and "other," always within historical and cultural contexts – that is, between traditions. Understanding, he maintained, cannot be separated from its historical and subjective dimensions, despite aspirations toward objectivity. Consequently, Gadamer argued against a fixed methodology for textual interpretation, as interpretation inherently resists the pursuit of purely objective knowledge.

Gadamer (1975) built upon Heidegger's thesis regarding the historicity of knowledge structure – that understanding is always preceded by prior understanding – and emphasized how existing categories of thought shape our acquisition of knowledge. For Gadamer, dialogue occurs between horizons of traditions, where a horizon represents "the range of vision that includes everything that can be seen from a particular vantage point" (p. 301). This horizon of tradition encompasses both historical perspectives and present situations, as well as the individual viewpoints embedded within them. Within these historical horizons lie what Gadamer termed "prejudices" – the prejudgments that shape our understanding.

For Gadamer, each person approaches interpretation with understandings rooted in their cultural tradition. These prejudices, rather than hindering understanding, actually enable it. The tradition's horizon provides the conceptual framework through which interpretation becomes possible, furnishing the conscious materials – the prejudices – through which we perceive and extract meaning. However, the interpreter must recognize both their own conceptual horizon and that of the other. Understanding emerges through openness to the text or to the other subject, while maintaining, rather than abandoning, one's preexisting judgments that arise from tradition.

Understanding, for Gadamer, is a process of "fusion of horizons." This means that genuine understanding emerges when we experience past concepts through present understanding in dialogue with a text or another subject. This fusion of horizons, while arising from dialogue, does not imply agreement; rather, it leads to an expansion of traditional horizons. It enables bridging between past and present horizons of tradition, and between different traditions, while maintaining awareness of their distinctiveness.

Gadamer maintained that understanding is not a finite achievement but an ongoing adaptation of meaning to concrete situations. Understanding does not uncover an objective truth in texts or encounters; rather, truth emerges dynamically through specific situations and participants. Yet, according to Gadamer, individuals within a specific cultural community remain bound by their culture's interpretive frameworks. This constraint prevents interpretation from falling into unlimited subjectivism (Mautner, 2000).

Traditions create both separation and connection: their different horizons establish distances between interpreter and text, past and present, subject and subject. Yet these horizons converge in the pursuit of understanding, existing within the shared context of human historical experience. While the horizon provides the interpretive materials – the prejudices – through which meaning emerges, the interpreter must recognize both their own horizon and that of the other to enable genuine dialogue. This fusion of horizons allows traditions to expand through engagement with one another while preserving their distinct identities.

Drawing from Gadamer's view of hermeneutics as fundamental to human understanding, we seek to establish a philosophical foundation for dialogue in psychotherapy integration. This addresses our central question: How can understanding emerge between psychotherapy schools that represent distinct and often opposing cultural traditions? Before applying Gadamer's ideas to advance dialogue between approaches, we will demonstrate that his philosophy already has significant resonance within mental health and psychotherapy, particularly psychoanalysis.

Gadamer's Dialogue in Psychoanalysis

In recent decades, Gadamer's ideas have increasingly influenced therapeutic discourse, particularly within the relational stream of psychoanalysis.

Mook (2010) argues that psychotherapy belongs to the human sciences rather than the natural sciences. She critiques the scientific paradigm and proposes hermeneutical phenomenological foundations for psychotherapy as a human science, drawing on Gadamer's hermeneutics to establish philosophical foundations for understanding reality and humanity. Gadamer's influence extends to psychotherapy research, particularly in qualitative studies where researchers must interpret their findings. Barak (2022) applies Gadamer's concepts to research findings, treating them as texts to be interpreted with cultural sensitivity and awareness of bias. In the context of therapeutic relationships, Wiercinski (2019) draws on Gadamer to argue that interpretive dialogue forms the foundation of the therapist-patient relationship. McWhorter (2021) further suggests that this dialogue aims to develop shared interpretive understanding, requiring openness to and awareness of cultural biases. This dialogical stance, according to McWhorter, enhances cultural sensitivity, empathy, and therapeutic alliance.

Gadamer's influence is most prominently evident in psychoanalytic writings, particularly within the relational perspective. Orange (2010) suggests that Gadamer's ideas provide post-Freudian psychoanalysts with a framework for critically examining conservative psychoanalytic theory and practice. The relational approach embodies this theoretical and practical shift in psychoanalysis through its emphasis on relationship systems in human psychology, both for development and for therapeutic understanding. This perspective has led to a reconceptualization of traditional elements including the therapeutic framework, analyst's role, treatment goals, and fundamentally, the nature and process of understanding in therapy. Central to this approach is the view that meaning emerges not from therapist authority but through collaborative meaning-making with the patient (Aron, 1996).

Mitchell and Aron (1999) conceptualize the analytic encounter as an intersubjective space – an interactive matrix where an analyst and a patient mutually influence each other, albeit not in an equal or symmetrical way. They argue that analysts do not simply observe and uncover psychoanalytic structures and patterns, but bring their own complex subjectivity, including their history, biases, and loyalties, to how they shape and understand the therapeutic process. Other theorists extend this view, arguing that the analyst's subjectivity is not a limitation to be overcome but rather an essential element that shapes interpersonal interaction and understanding in therapy (Hoffman, 1983; Renik, 1993; Stern, 2013).

Drawing on Gadamerian hermeneutics, Stern (2003) challenges the notion of therapist as blank slate, arguing that interpretive truth emerges through interpersonal and cultural contexts. Orange (2002) extends this perspective, emphasizing that meaning production transcends the therapeutic dyad and is embedded in broader cultural contexts. Stern (1991, 2013) further argues that effective understanding requires therapists to recognize their own preconceptions, which both facilitate and potentially impede understanding without openness to questioning. For these scholars, the analytic encounter occurs fundamentally through language (Orange, 2003; Renik, 1993; Stern, 1983); as Gadamer argued, both the encounter itself and its meaning are mediated by language.

Writers from the relational perspective in psychoanalysis have consistently drawn upon Gadamer's philosophy to ground their theoretical positions. This perspective reconceptualizes psychoanalysis as an interpersonal process shaped by professional, cultural, and social contexts, where understanding emerges through shared dialogue. As Eaton (1998) succinctly states, "At bottom, therapy, on this reading, is a mutually interpretative endeavor" (p. 424). Building on this understanding, Clarke (1997) emphasizes the fundamental connection between relational psychoanalysis and hermeneutics:

> The truth is that one cannot develop a decent relational psychoanalytic model without also addressing how people know one another and the world, or how we should best talk about this relationship; and this is helped enormously by philosophy, pragmatist or otherwise. If the principles of philosophical hermeneutics are accepted (or deemed useful), as I will argue they should be, then we should also consider granting universal reach to their accompanying epistemological

claims. This is the radical bottom-line of Gadamer's position, and one of the reasons he deserves continued attention from psychoanalytic theorists – whether to incorporate, to modify, or to argue against.

(p. 10)

These writers demonstrate commitment to fostering understanding within the therapeutic relationship and promoting authentic dialogue, despite the inherent gaps created by each participant's historical subjectivity. While this commitment reflects the fundamental aim of all psychotherapeutic approaches – helping the patient – it is noteworthy that the psychoanalytic school, like other therapeutic approaches, has not actively pursued dialogue with other psychotherapeutic schools to enhance treatment effectiveness. This reluctance may stem from what we discussed earlier – the perceived threat to professional-cultural identity and fear of its destabilization. However, just as psychoanalysis has embraced Gadamer's ideas for dialogue with patients, we propose extending these principles to facilitate dialogue with other approaches, particularly its historical rival, CBT.

Gadamer's Dialogue in Psychotherapy Integration

In this section, we present Gadamer's hermeneutic principles to demonstrate how understanding can emerge through dialogue between psychotherapeutic schools and to explore the potential meanings of such dialogue. While our presentation divides these principles into distinct categories, we acknowledge this division's artificial nature. Gadamer himself argues against systematic methods for understanding texts or for hermeneutical understanding in general, and these principles are inherently interconnected, emerging from and existing in relationship with one another. Nevertheless, this organizational framework allows us to identify key conditions for meaningful dialogue. Importantly, these conditions suggest not merely theoretical possibilities but practical applications for therapeutic discourse.

Understanding as Application

Given the intermediate position in which hermeneutics operates, it follows that its work is not to develop a procedure of understanding, but to clarify the conditions in which understanding takes place.

(Gadamer, 1975, p. 295)

Gadamer (1975) shifts focus from developing methodological procedures to examining the fundamental conditions that make understanding possible. His concern lies not in how to construct a systematic approach to understanding but in identifying what enables understanding to occur at all.

According to Gadamer, meaning emerges through three inseparable and simultaneous processes: understanding, interpretation, and application. Understanding and interpretation are mutually constitutive – each emerges through and shapes the other. Application represents the actualization of understanding within specific historical and cultural contexts. These three elements – interpretation, understanding, and application – form an inseparable unity in the creation of meaning. When we understand something through dialogue with others, we engage in self-understanding through interpretation that is always applied to our current context.

Through this framework, Gadamer offers practical insights without imposing a rigid scientific method. While science aims to strip the experience of its historical and subjective elements in pursuit of objectivity, Gadamer argues that such reduction distorts the very nature of human understanding. His concern lies with truth and knowledge as they emerge through lived experience, rather than with verifying an objective reality. While Gadamer's hermeneutics does not prescribe a specific method, it offers conditions for understanding through dialogue.

In the context of psychotherapy integration, this raises a fundamental question about the conditions necessary for such dialogue: How can therapists from different schools engage in genuine exchange that enables them to understand both the other approach and themselves a new?

To explore these conditions, let us consider a conference on anxiety disorders where therapists from different approaches present their work. If we focus on representatives from psychoanalytic and cognitive-behavioral schools, several questions emerge: What would enable them to truly listen to each other? What would allow them to understand something meaningful about each other's approaches and the clinical material being discussed? Moreover, what could facilitate new insights about their own approaches through this exchange? These questions point to the fundamental challenge of creating conditions for meaningful dialogue between different therapeutic traditions.

Understanding as Involvement

To understand it does not mean primarily to reason one's way back into the past, but to have a present involvement in what is.

(Gadamer, 1975, p. 393)

For Gadamer (1975), understanding begins when we are addressed by someone or something that calls for our attention. This understanding requires active personal involvement; without willingness to engage, genuine understanding cannot emerge. This principle applies whether we are engaging in dialogue with a text or with another person – in both cases, there must be readiness to understand the matter at hand.

Fouché and Smit (1996) characterize Gadamer's approach as dialogue based on "goodwill." This involves openness to the other and recognition that the other has something meaningful to contribute. Such dialogue requires mutual willingness: the self must be ready to receive the other's address, and the other must be willing to engage. However, Fouché and Smit emphasize that this "goodwill" is directed not primarily toward the dialogue partner but toward the subject matter itself and the new understanding that can emerge through dialogue. This "goodwill" thus represents an ethical commitment to knowledge itself. As Gadamer (1975) notes, "Since here the object of experience is a person, this kind of experience is a moral phenomenon – as is the knowledge acquired through experience, the understanding of the other person" (p. 352).

Therapists' readiness to engage in dialogue can emerge from their shared commitment to helping patients. This active involvement is essential; without such willingness, no genuine understanding can emerge. When psychoanalytic and cognitive-behavioral therapists participate in dialogue, as in our example, what matters is not primarily their desire to understand each other's approach but their shared commitment to understanding the subject matter itself – the effective treatment of anxiety disorders.

Understanding as Content-Focused

> Something is placed in the center, as the Greeks say, which the partners in dialogue both share, and concerning which they can exchange ideas with one another.
>
> (Gadamer, 1975, p. 371)

For Gadamer (1975), the focus of dialogue lies in understanding the content being discussed rather than understanding the speaker themselves. Whether interpreting a text or engaging in conversation, the primary aim is not to understand the author or interlocutor but to understand the subject matter in new ways. Understanding emerges through shared engagement with a specific topic that stands at the center of the dialogue.

This principle can facilitate dialogue between psychotherapeutic schools by focusing attention on shared professional concerns. Such dialogue might address theoretical understanding, clinical practice, or research methodology. By focusing on the subject matter rather than on defending or critiquing particular schools, practitioners may find their usual defensive stances softening.

Let's return to our example and imagine a cognitive-behavioral therapist presenting anxiety disorder treatment at a conference. The psychoanalytic therapist is asked to respond in the subsequent discussion. However, the request is not for the psychoanalytic therapist to justify the cognitive-behavioral approach, explain why it works, or convert to that approach. Instead, the psychoanalytic therapist is asked to discuss the proposed topic, the presented content, with questions like: How do I understand what worked in the treatment? How can I understand what helped the patient? How can these understandings serve therapy in general? When the object of understanding is not the speaker – the cognitive-behavioral therapist or CBT – but the topic being discussed – treatment of social anxiety – the psychoanalytic therapist can engage without raising barriers of resistance and antagonism.

However, while therapists' goodwill reflects their ethical stance and shared concern for patients' well-being, it would be naive to assume that this commitment alone can overcome professional barriers. As discussed earlier, therapists' attachments to their professional-cultural identities often lead them to avoid dialogue that might challenge these identities. Yet Gadamer's thinking offers insights into addressing this challenge as well.

Understanding as Rooted in Tradition

We are always situated within traditions, and this is no objectifying process – i.e., we do not conceive of what tradition says as something other, something alien. It is always part of us, a model or exemplar, a kind of cognizance that our later historical judgment would hardly regard as a kind of knowledge but as the most ingenuous affinity with tradition.

(Gadamer, 1975, p. 283)

While we have discussed involvement as a willingness that stems from goodwill to engage in dialogue about shared topics, Gadamer (1975) points to another crucial dimension. For him, involvement necessarily includes engagement from within one's historical tradition. This emphasizes the inherently historical and subjective nature of understanding – the interpreter cannot step outside their traditional frame-work but always understands from within it.

This tradition functions as an a priori condition of understanding, providing the fundamental materials that construct a person's identity: their perceptions, beliefs, values, and practices. In the context of psychotherapy, such tradition shapes the therapist's professional identity – whether psychoanalytic or cognitive-behavioral – through a distinctive set of theoretical understandings and clinical practices. While psychotherapeutic traditions have evolved over time, incorporating various developments and streams of thought, their core principles continue to serve as foundational anchors:

For example, classic psychoanalytic tradition (Freud, 1913/1989, 1915/1989, 1916) centers on the conflict between drives of sexuality and aggression originating in the id and the restraining forces of the superego. This intrapsychic conflict manifests through ego defense mechanisms, such as repression of forbidden material into the unconscious, potentially resulting in psychopathological symptoms. While later developments in psychoanalysis shifted away from drive theory, the concept of unconscious conflict remained central to the tradition. Another focus in therapy is the transference relationship between a therapist and a patient, where the patient projects internalized early life figures onto the therapeutic relationship. Accordingly, psychoanalytic practice typically focuses on these unconscious (interpersonal and intrapersonal) processes, making central use of free associations and interpretations to bring the unconscious to consciousness and promote insight as a key therapeutic goal.

In contrast, cognitive-behavioral tradition (Knapp & Beck, 2008) emphasizes how early learning experiences shape core beliefs (schemas) about the self, others, and the world. These core beliefs, which function as mental structures organizing information, often operate outside consciousness. When triggered by specific present events, they generate automatic thoughts that are typically more accessible to awareness. Negative early experiences can lead to negative schemas that produce distorted automatic thoughts about life events, resulting in behaviors that reinforce these core beliefs and manifest in various forms of psychopathology. Consequently, CBT focuses on identifying and addressing factors that maintain symptoms in the present – including environmental triggers, maladaptive thinking patterns, and problematic behaviors. Treatment typically involves identifying, challenging, and modifying the cognitions and behaviors that perpetuate psychological difficulties.

Do these fundamentally different traditions preclude mutual understanding? For Gadamer, quite the opposite is true: understanding occurs precisely through and because of tradition, not in spite of it. He views the tension between the familiar and the unfamiliar not as an unbridgeable gap, but as the very condition that makes understanding possible. This perspective suggests that even when psychotherapeutic schools represent distinctly different traditions, understanding remains possible. The movement between different traditions' horizons – whether between past and present, or between self and other – does not require abandoning one's familiar ground but rather proceeds from within it, making understanding of the other possible.

Understanding, therefore, emerges through mediation – between present situation and historical tradition, between interpreter and text, between self and other. In our conference example, therapists engage not only with the immediate discussion of anxiety disorders but also through their respective therapeutic traditions. Their capacity to understand new perspectives arises precisely from within their own traditional horizons.

Tradition as an a priori condition for understanding suggests that while it allows for involvement in dialogue and understanding, it will always be limited by it. We wish to argue that this maintains a dialectical tension that can allow for openness to the subject for representatives of the psychotherapeutic schools. On the one hand, the goodwill to participate in dialogue with the other school. On the other hand, the limits of tradition can also negate the threat to their professional identity.

Understanding Through Prejudice

> Prejudices are biases of our openness to the world. They are simply conditions whereby we experience something – whereby what we encounter says something to us.

> (Gadamer, 1966, p. 9)

For Gadamer (1975), "prejudice" refers to categories of thought shaped by historical and cultural processes. Rather than viewing prejudice as an error to be eliminated, he sees it as an essential foundation for understanding, embedded within tradition's horizon. These prejudices constitute our way of being in and understanding the world – they precede and make possible all subsequent understanding.

Bernstein (2008) notes that prejudice within tradition's horizon simultaneously enables openness to dialogue while establishing boundaries that preserve tradition. Thus, prejudice serves both as a condition for understanding and as a framework that defines its limits.

The psychotherapeutic traditions we discussed – psychoanalytic and cognitive-behavioral – each operate from distinct preconceptions about fundamental questions: the nature of healthy development, the origins of psychopathology, the goals of therapy, appropriate therapeutic practices, criteria for successful treatment, the therapist's role, and valid research methodologies. These prejudices emerge from theoretical training within each school's tradition, shaped further by personal and cultural histories. While such prejudices might seem to impede understanding between schools, Gadamer's perspective suggests that they may actually enable meaningful dialogue and mutual understanding.

Thus, in the encounter described in the example, the preconceptions of each of the participants – the prejudices that may seem like an obstacle – are what will allow for understanding of the treatment of anxiety and what worked in it. At the same time, these prejudices also limit this openness and thus preserve the boundaries of the tradition while expanding it. In such an encounter, there is no danger of assimilation or loss of professional-cultural identity. Yet the question arises: What is required in order to hold a productive dialogue? A dialogue that will maintain the tension between openness and limits and will not be thwarted by prejudice.

Understanding as a Dialogue of Question and Answer

> In dialogue spoken language – in the process of question and answer, giving and taking, talking at cross purposes and seeing each other's point – performs the communication of meaning that, with respect to the written tradition, is the task of hermeneutics.
>
> (Gadamer, 1975, p. 361)

Dialogue is necessary, according to Gadamer (1975), because the horizons of each participant, whether text or subject, differ from one another. This difference shapes the encounter both between interpreter and text, and between subjects, as encounters marked by fundamental alienation and strangeness. To overcome this alienation that could block understanding, Gadamer conceptualizes interpretation as inherently dialogical, similar to conversation between people.

For Gadamer, dialogue represents the art of questioning and the search for truth. Led by openness, dialogue manifests in the model of question and answer. The question forms the essence of dialogue and enables its existence only when it remains open to the various possibilities that may arise in the answer:

> To ask a question means to bring into the open. The openness of what is in question consists in the fact that the answer is not settled...Every true question requires this openness. Without it, it is basically no more than an apparent question.
>
> (Gadamer, 1975, p. 357)

Openness in dialogue involves willingness to examine one's prejudices and to view the subject matter from the perspective of the other's horizon. Gadamer suggests that rather than arguing, participants should give weight to each other's opinions and actively seek the strengths in opposing viewpoints. This requires both awareness of one's prejudices and readiness to examine whether these prejudices block the understanding or whether they can be examined, reflected upon, and criticized in ways that renew their meaning.

Consider our example of dialogue between psychotherapeutic schools, where a psychoanalytic therapist attempts to understand anxiety disorder treatment through a cognitive-behavioral therapist's case presentation. This encounter raises meaningful questions: How do these different traditions understand the problem's development and maintenance? How do they conceptualize therapeutic methods and mechanisms of change? What do they identify as the challenges and limitations of their respective approaches?

Such questions arise not merely as formal inquiries but from a genuine desire to understand the effectiveness of the presented treatment and gain new insights. This understanding necessarily emerges from within each participant's therapeutic tradition and its inherent prejudices. The process requires both awareness of these prejudices and careful examination of how they might facilitate or hinder understanding. True dialogue transcends simple exchange of opinions, demanding authentic curiosity and openness to move between established knowledge and new understanding. In this way, the process of understanding maintains tradition's boundaries while allowing its horizons to expand.

The structure of question and answer characteristic of this dialogical process creates a framework for understanding between traditions. This dynamic process occurs within the medium of language, which enables both the dialogical exchange itself and the emergence of new meanings.

Understanding as Located Within Language

Language is the universal medium in which understanding occurs.

(Gadamer, 1975, p. 390)

According to Gadamer (1975), the encounter between interpreter and text, or between person and other, occurs within language, deals with language, and finds its meaning through language. Language serves as the medium through which we live and understand our world at every moment. For Gadamer, language represents the essential mode of human existence – being, thinking, understanding, and language are inseparable. Language is not merely a tool we use but the very space in which we live and understand. It contains within it the horizons of culture, personal and social history, tradition, and prejudice. These historical and subjective dimensions, together with the linguistic framework, form the foundation for the ongoing dynamic process of understanding.

Returning to our conference example, where psychoanalytic and cognitive-behavioral therapists present their approaches to treating anxiety, we encounter a fundamental question: How is understanding possible when each school speaks such a different language? Classical psychoanalysis expresses itself through concepts like the unconscious, drives, intrapsychic conflict, defense mechanisms, transference and countertransference, and repetition compulsion. CBT, in contrast, employs terms like core beliefs, schemas, automatic thoughts, and behavioral patterns. If understanding occurs through language, and if language itself carries cultural traditions and prejudices, how can meaningful dialogue emerge between such distinct therapeutic languages?

First, Gadamer argues that the very need to convey meaning between languages underscores the centrality of language in understanding. This transfer of meaning occurs through *translation*, where meaning is not simply copied but interpreted. For Gadamer (1975), "The translation process fundamentally contains the whole secret of how human beings come to an understanding of the world and communicate with each other" (p. 552). When we seek to understand something, we translate from one tradition's language into another tradition's language. This translation enables understanding from within the horizons of the tradition seeking to understand. For Gadamer, while translation should convey what the original text (or speaker) discusses, it inevitably produces new meaning rather than merely copying existing meaning.

According to this principle, translation between languages is essential for meaning and understanding to emerge. How, then, might such translation occur between different psychotherapeutic languages in our conference example?

Consider the cognitive-behavioral therapist presenting his work with anxiety disorders. He describes treating a patient with social anxiety, explaining how therapy involves monitoring specific situations where the patient experiences distress (for instance, speaking in class). The therapist details how he identifies, together with the patient, the thoughts that trigger anxiety ("I am not smart," "others will think I am stupid and will mock me"), and the resulting avoidance behaviors aimed at reducing anxiety (such as avoiding class participation). At the cognitive level, the therapist describes identifying the source of automatic thoughts in core beliefs (schemas), using techniques like the "downward arrow" method and Socratic questioning to explore the meaning behind each response. Through this process, the patient and the therapist uncover a chain of beliefs: speaking up will lead others to think the patient is not smart, this perceived lack of intelligence will lead to social rejection, and this rejection confirms the patient's sense of worthlessness and isolation. The therapist links these core beliefs ("I am worthless," "I will remain alone") and their resulting automatic thoughts to early experiences with critical, rigid, and contemptuous parents who showed preference for a sibling. Importantly, the therapist emphasizes that the goal is not merely achieving this insight, but understanding how these core beliefs, automatic thoughts, and avoidant behaviors perpetuate the patient's sense of worthlessness and isolation. The therapist describes the therapeutic process: challenging these cognitions through examining evidence for and against them, developing alternative thoughts ("I understand the subject," "people are interested in what I say"), and creating opportunities for new learning experiences through exposure.

As this case is presented, the psychoanalytic therapist in the audience encounters a conceptual world that may seem foreign or even questionable from his perspective. Yet this raises crucial questions: How can he understand what is actually occurring in this anxiety treatment? How can he make sense of the patient's reported improvement? What might this treatment approach reveal about working with anxiety disorders?

Let us explore how understanding might emerge through translation between these therapeutic languages. The psychoanalytic therapist might understand the patient's distress by translating it into his familiar concepts: unconscious conflict (involving the need for others, fear of rejection, and defensive avoidance of psychic pain). He might understand schemas as analogous to internalized mental representations or internalized objects of parental figures. Similarly, he could interpret the cognitive focus on identifying distress sources (how early experiences shape schemas that generate anxiety-producing automatic thoughts) as parallel to the psychoanalytic process of bringing unconscious material into consciousness. Building on this process of translation, the psychoanalytic therapist might also understand the monitoring of events in CBT as analogous to working with free associations. Moreover, he can interpret the collaborative therapeutic relationship as a form of corrective emotional experience, where transference processes enable the internalization of more beneficial parental objects.

Through such translation – from the presented language to his own therapeutic framework – the therapist can achieve genuine understanding of the treatment without needing to either reject or fully adopt the cognitive-behavioral approach. He can grasp how and why the treatment works because he understands it through his own therapeutic lens while maintaining focus on the central question: What helps in treating anxiety? This highlights that the goal of understanding is not to comprehend the other approach per se but to understand what facilitates effective treatment of anxiety disorders.

According to Gadamer, translation between languages – as in our example of psychoanalysis and CBT – represents just one possible outcome of dialogue. His hermeneutics suggests another possibility: the emergence of a *new language* through dialogue itself. While participants begin with their distinct therapeutic languages, their dialogue about a shared subject matter can generate new ways of understanding and speaking about therapeutic processes. This creates not just interpretations of existing ideas but novel conceptual frameworks.

Such a language can develop through trans-theoretical concepts such as schemas or unconscious processes. Mares (2022) suggests that identifying trans-theoretical structures common to different approaches provides a form of "translation" that enables productive exchange and integration while preserving each approach's distinct identity. For example, Mares points to unconscious processes as a trans-theoretical concept shared by psychoanalysis and CBT, bridging concepts such as core beliefs (schemas) and internalized mental representations. Similarly, Moorey (2010) suggests that schema itself can serve as a trans-theoretical structure, providing a common language through which psychoanalysis and CBT can communicate.

Through this lens, for instance, transference in psychoanalysis can be understood as a specific relationship schema operating in the therapeutic interaction.

The integrative movement in psychotherapy exemplifies a unique developmental path. While maintaining its fundamental goal of fostering dialogue between different therapeutic traditions, it has simultaneously evolved to develop its own conceptual frameworks. This includes the creation of trans-theoretical concepts and the identification of common factors across approaches (Norcross & Alexander, 2019). This development reflects not an attempt to establish a separate tradition but rather an effort to create bridging languages that can facilitate meaningful dialogue between existing traditions.

These attempts at translation and creation of new therapeutic language raise a fundamental question: What emerges from these processes of understanding? How does this understanding, whether through translation or new conceptual frameworks, transform our therapeutic knowledge?

Understanding as a Fusion of Horizons

It is the historically experienced consciousness that, by renouncing the chimera of perfect enlightenment, is open to the experience of history. We described its realization as the fusion of the horizons of understanding, which is what mediates between the text and its interpreter.

(Gadamer, 1975, p. 370)

For Gadamer (1975), understanding emerges when the historical horizons of different traditions meet in the present dialogue. This meeting occurs when we move from our own horizon toward the horizon of another tradition, while simultaneously maintaining our own perspective. It is precisely this ability to extend beyond our horizon while remaining grounded within it that enables meaningful dialogue and understanding. In this process, each historical tradition's perspective engages with the other in the present moment, creating a dynamic interplay between past and present, between self and other. Understanding becomes possible through this simultaneous holding of multiple perspectives – reaching toward the other's horizon while remaining anchored in our own.

This process results in what Gadamer terms a "fusion of horizons," expanding the horizons of the tradition from which we began our understanding. However, this fusion is not a simple merging or blending of different perspectives. Drawing on Hegel's dialectical thinking (2018 [1807]), Gadamer describes how meaning emerges through the movement from one tradition's horizon toward another's, and then back again. When we return to our own tradition after engaging with another's horizon, we achieve a more complex understanding of our own position. As Makkreel (1997) notes, Gadamer's conception, inspired by Hegel, describes an internal process of meaning-making that leads to self-development through engagement with the other.

The purpose of dialogue between psychotherapeutic schools, therefore, is neither to validate one approach over another nor to achieve consensus but to create a space where each tradition's perspective can expand and deepen while maintaining its distinct identity. Through encounter with another school, each approach can discover new meanings in its own theories and practices – meanings that become visible precisely through engagement with a different tradition.

Returning to our conference example, this process of understanding enables the psychoanalytic therapist to expand his traditional framework in several ways (though we will focus here on the psychoanalytic perspective, similar expansion is possible for the cognitive-behavioral therapist). Through this understanding, he can expand his interpretive approach to recognize connections between learning processes and the perception of self and other. He can broaden the boundaries of his practice to include greater focus on present situations that arouse anxiety. Moreover, he can expand his understanding of therapeutic positioning to see how exposure work might constitute a response to deprivation and serve as a corrective emotional experience. This does not suggest that such therapeutic elements were absent before; rather, the dialogue offers an opportunity to understand existing practices from a new perspective. Through this process of understanding, the therapist not only gains new insights about therapeutic work but also expands the boundaries of his own therapeutic tradition.

Govrin (2019) provides a useful framework for understanding such development. He distinguishes between two types of psychoanalytic innovation: "first-order" innovation, which characterized canonical theory through new discoveries about the psyche, development, transference, and psychopathology; and "second-order" innovation, which emerges in recent decades through challenging methodological and philosophical assumptions without replacing existing theory. This second-order innovation represents a new "sensitivity" that practitioners integrate into their existing framework. The fusion of horizons that Gadamer describes, and which we explore in this chapter, can facilitate precisely this kind of innovation – not undermining tradition but enriching it through new sensitivities that emerge from dialogue with other approaches.

Understanding as Construction

> The horizon is, rather, something into which we move and that moves with us. Horizons change for a person who is moving. Thus, the horizon of the past, out of which all human life lives and which exists in the form of tradition, is always in motion. The surrounding horizon is not set in motion by historical consciousness. But in it this motion becomes aware of itself.
>
> (Gadamer, 1975, p. 303)

The fusion of horizons has a historical dimension, wherein the past horizons of one tradition seek to understand something through the past horizons of another tradition in the present moment. The past serves as the ground from which present understanding becomes possible. Yet tradition is not merely a static force shaping our present perception; rather, it develops and transforms as we engage in the act of understanding through it. Each act of understanding in the present, mediating the past, contributes to tradition's continuous development.

Thus, understanding through the fusion of horizons mediates not only between different traditions but also between past and present within each tradition. As a result, it can be seen that tradition, for Gadamer (1975), is never static; understanding emerges not as the revelation of absolute truth but as its dynamic construction. Meaning does not reside passively in the object of interpretation awaiting discovery, but rather emerges through an ongoing process of engagement. Each interpretive encounter produces understanding anew through the active connection between the interpreter and the object of understanding.

While interpretation as an existential act is boundless, reflecting history's continuous motion, this does not imply pure subjectivity where each person generates entirely individual meanings. As previously discussed, tradition and prejudice both enable and constrain understanding. For Gadamer, understanding occurs within traditional horizons – it can expand these horizons but cannot transcend them entirely. The subject matter itself, together with the interpreter's tradition, provides boundaries that prevent understanding from dissolving into pure relativism. Thus, while multiple interpretive possibilities exist, they are not unlimited. As Gadamer (1975) emphasizes,

> Now, the fact is that meanings represent a fluid multiplicity of possibilities (in comparison to the agreement presented by a language and a vocabulary), but within this multiplicity of what can be thought – i.e., of what a reader can find meaningful and hence expect to find – not everything is possible.
>
> (p. 271)

Here we encounter another central dialectic in Gadamer's hermeneutics: understanding is simultaneously ongoing and bounded. On one side, understanding is never complete but occurs through recurring hermeneutic circles, with each encounter generating new meanings. On the other side, our embeddedness in historical tradition means that all understanding remains inherently limited and partial (Gadamer, 2006).

Hence, the understandings that emerge among practitioners from different psychotherapeutic schools (as in our conference example on anxiety treatment) represent not fixed truths but products of joint creation, shaped by the participants, time, and context. The dialogue between schools opens up various creative possibilities rather than leading to final conclusions. Each encounter between psychotherapeutic schools – whether through texts or direct interaction – carries the potential for dynamic development of traditions and enrichment with new meanings, while preserving traditional boundaries. This potential can be realized when conditions for genuine dialogue are met.

Final Conclusions

> The ongoing dialogue permits no final conclusion. It would be a poor hermeneuticist who thought he could have, or had to have, the last word.
>
> (Gadamer, 1975, p. 581)

This fundamental principle reminds us that our interpretation of dialogue through Gadamer's hermeneutical framework remains open to continuous development. With this understanding, we offer conclusions that emerge from our present engagement with these ideas.

While Gadamer's hermeneutical thought has been productively applied to understanding the therapeutic encounter between the analyst and the patient, its potential for facilitating dialogue between different therapeutic schools remains largely unexplored. This chapter proposes extending Gadamer's framework to enable meaningful interaction between distinct psychotherapeutic traditions. Establishing this dialogical foundation is crucial for the integration movement's emphasis on psychotherapy integration as an ongoing process of dialogue between diverse therapeutic traditions.

Where previous integration efforts often emphasized commonalities between approaches, our application of Gadamer's hermeneutics suggests that meaningful dialogue can emerge precisely through engagement with differences. Such an approach, we argue, can foster openness to alternative perspectives while preserving the integrity of each tradition, enabling mutual enrichment without compromising distinctive identities. This dialogue between therapeutic schools not only serves to vitalize each approach but advances the entire field, while maintaining our central purpose: enhancing therapeutic effectiveness for our patients.

Building upon these theoretical insights, Gadamer's hermeneutics expands the philosophical-epistemological framework presented in this book, illuminating possibilities for meaningful encounters between psychotherapeutic traditions. The dialogical hermeneutics of Gadamer emerges here not as an abstract theoretical framework or ethical ideal but as a pragmatic and implementable approach to professional relationships.

Productive professional dialogue becomes possible when practitioners feel secure in their professional and cultural identity. When therapists perceive their tradition as protected rather than threatened, they can engage in open discourse with colleagues from different theoretical orientations. Through mutual recognition and respect of each tradition's distinctive identity, while understanding how tradition both enables and bounds dialogue, practitioners can maintain both their uniqueness and openness to other perspectives.

When psychotherapeutic schools engage in active dialogue – exploring shared concerns, examining assumptions, and considering alternative perspectives – new understandings emerge that neither could achieve in isolation. Such dialogical encounters enable a fusion of horizons that expand understanding and promotes innovation. Each tradition discovers new dimensions of self-understanding through engagement with the other, as Gadamer (1966) articulates: "Only the support of familiar and common understanding makes possible the venture into the alien, the lifting up of something out of the alien, and thus the broadening and enrichment of our own experience of the world" (p. 15).

We propose that understanding Gadamer's insights regarding the conditions for dialogue and the nature of understanding – as simultaneously preserving and developing tradition – can facilitate meaningful encounters between clinicians from different therapeutic approaches. Future efforts of the integration movement might productively focus on creating dialogical spaces where traditions can both maintain their integrity and evolve through engagement with others. These encounters can foster a dynamic tradition that extends beyond historical inheritance to become an ongoing creative process. Through such dialogue, traditions not only gain insight into alternative approaches but discover deeper dimensions of their own theoretical foundations and clinical practices, enriching rather than abandoning their heritage.

References

Aron, L. (1996). *A meeting of minds: Mutuality in psychoanalysis.* Hillsdale, NJ: Analytic Press, Inc.

Barak, A. (2022). Fusing horizons in qualitative research: Gadamer and cultural resonances. *Qualitative Research in Psychology, 19*(3), 768–783.

Bernstein, R. J. (2008). The conversation that never happened (Gadamer/Derrida). *The Review of Metaphysics, 61*(3), 577–603.

Clarke, B. H. (1997). Hermeneutics and the "relational" turn: Schafer, Ricoeur, Gadamer, and the nature of psychoanalytic subjectivity. *Psychoanalysis and Contemporary Thought, 20*(1), 3–68.

Eaton, J. (1998). Gadamer: Psychotherapy as conversation. *European Journal of Psychotherapy & Counselling, 1*(3), 421–433.

Fouché, H. L., & Smit, D. J. (1996). Inviting a dialogue on 'Dialogue'. *Scriptura: Journal for Biblical, Theological and Contextual Hermeneutics, 57,* 79–102.

Freud, S. (1913/1989). On beginning the treatment. In P. Gay (Ed.), *The Freud reader* (pp. 363–378). New York, NY: W.W. Norton.

Freud, S. (1915/1989). The unconscious. In P. Gay (Ed.), *The Freud reader* (pp. 572–584). New York, NY: W.W. Norton.

Freud, S. (1916). Introductory lectures on psychoanalysis. In J. Strachey (Trans. & Ed.), *The standard edition of the complete psychological works of Sigmund Freud* (Vol. 16, pp. 327–343). London: Hogarth Press.

Gadamer, H. G. (1966/1976). The universality of the hermeneutical problem. In D. E. Linge (Ed.), *Philosophical hermeneutics* (pp. 3–17). Berkeley, CA: University of California Press.

Gadamer, H. G. (1975/2004). *Truth and method* (J. Weinsheimer & D. G. Marshall, Trans.; 2nd Rev. Ed.). New York, NY: Continuum.

Gadamer, H. G. (2006). *A century of philosophy: Hans Georg Gadamer in conversation with Riccardo Dottori.* New York, NY: Bloomsbury Publishing USA.]

Goldfried, M. R. (2019). Obtaining consensus in psychotherapy: What holds us back? *American Psychologist, 74*(4), 484–496.

Goldfried, M. R., Pachankis, J. E., & Bell, A. C. (2005). A history of psychotherapy integration. In J. C. Norcross & M. R. Goldfried (Eds.), *Handbook of psychotherapy integration* (2nd ed., pp. 24–60). New York, NY: Oxford University Press.

Goldfried, M. R., Pachankis, J. E., & Goodwin, B. J. (2019) A history of psychotherapy integration. In J. C. Norcross & M. R. Goldfried (Eds.), *Handbook of psychotherapy integration* (3rd ed., pp. 28–63). New York, NY: Oxford University Press.

Govrin, A. (2019). Facts and sensibilities: What is a psychoanalytic innovation? *Frontiers in Psychology, 10*, Article 1781. https://doi.org/10.3389/fpsyg.2019.01781

Hegel, G. W. F. (1807/2018). *The phenomenology of spirit* (M. Inwood, Trans.). Oxford: Oxford University Press.

Heidegger, M. (1962). *Being and time*. Oxford: Blackwell Publishing.

Hoffman, I. Z. (1983). The patient as interpreter of the analyst's experience. *Contemporary Psychoanalysis, 19*(3), 389–422.

Knapp, P., & Beck, A. T. (2008). Cognitive therapy: Foundations, conceptual models, applications and research. *Brazilian Journal of Psychiatry, 30*(Suppl. 2), S54–S64.

McWhorter, M. R. (2021). Gadamer's philosophical hermeneutics and the formation of mental health professionals. *Journal of Theoretical and Philosophical Psychology, 41*(3), 187–207.

Makkreel, R. A. (1997). Gadamer and the problem of how to relate Kant and Hegel to hermeneutics. *Laval théologique et philosophique, 53*(1), 151–166.

Mares, L. (2022). Unconscious processes in psychoanalysis, CBT, and schema therapy. *Journal of Psychotherapy Integration, 32*(4), 443–452.

Mautner, M. (2000). Hans-Georg Gadamer and the law. *Tel Aviv University Law Review, 23*, 367–419.

Miller, R. B. (1992). Introduction to the philosophy of clinical psychology. In R. B. Miller (Ed.), *The restoration of dialogue: Readings in the philosophy of clinical psychology* (pp. 1–27). Washington, DC: American Psychological Association.

Mitchell, S. A., & Aron, L. (1999). Preface. In S. A. Mitchell & L. Aron (Eds.), *Relational psychoanalysis: The emergence of a tradition* (pp. ix–xx). Hillsdale, NJ: Analytic Press.

Mook, B. (2010). Hermeneutic phenomenology and psychotherapy. *Les Collectifs du Cirps, 1*, 209–222.

Moorey, S. (2010). Cognitive behaviour therapy and psychoanalysis. In A. Lemma & M. Patrick (Eds.), *Off the couch* (pp. 210–227). London: Routledge.

Norcross, J. C., & Alexander, E. F. (2019). A primer on psychotherapy integration. In J. C. Norcross & M. R. Goldfried (Eds.), *Handbook of psychotherapy integration* (3rd ed., pp. 3–27). New York, NY: Oxford University Press.

Orange, D. M. (2002). There is no outside: Empathy and authenticity in psychoanalysis process. *Psychoanalytic Psychology, 19*(4), 686–700.

Orange, D. M. (2003). Why language matters to psychoanalysis. *Psychoanalytic Dialogues, 13*(1), 77–103.

Orange, D. M. (2010). *Thinking for clinicians: Philosophical resources for contemporary psychoanalysis and the humanistic psychotherapies*. New York, NY: Routledge.

Peri Herzovich, Y., & Govrin, A. (2021). Psychoanalysis and CBT: From rivalry to hospitality in psychotherapy integration. *British Journal of Psychotherapy, 37*(2), 244–262.

Renik, O. (1993). Analytic interaction: Conceptualizing technique in light of the analyst's irreducible subjectivity. *The Psychoanalytic Quarterly, 62*(4), 553–571.

Safran, J. D., & Messer, S. B. (1997). Psychotherapy integration: A postmodern critique. *Clinical Psychology: Science & Practice, 4*(2), 140–152.

Stern, H. H. (1983). *Fundamental concepts of language teaching*. Oxford: Oxford University Press.

Stern, D. B. (1991). A philosophy for the embedded analyst: Gadamer's hermeneutics and the social paradigm of psychoanalysis. *Contemporary Psychoanalysis, 27*(1), 51–80.

Stern, D. B. (2003). *Unformulated Experience: From dissociation to imagination in psychoanalysis*. New York, NY: Psychology Press.

Stern, D. B. (2013). Psychotherapy is an emergent process: In favor of acknowledging hermeneutics and against the privileging of systematic empirical research. *Psychoanalytic Dialogues, 23*(1), 102–115.

Stricker, G. (2010). A second look at psychotherapy integration. *Journal of Psychotherapy Integration, 20*(4), 397–405.

Wachtel, P. L. (2010). Psychotherapy integration and integrative psychotherapy: Process or product? *Journal of Psychotherapy Integration, 20*(4), 406–416.

Wachtel, P. L. (2018). Pathways to progress for integrative psychotherapy: Perspectives on practice and research. *Journal of Psychotherapy Integration, 28*(2), 202–212.

Wachtel, P. L., & Goldfried, M. R. (2005). A critical dialogue on psychotherapy integration. In J. C. Norcross & M. R. Goldfried (Eds.), *Handbook of psychotherapy integration* (2nd ed., pp. 496–504). New York, NY : Oxford University Press.

Wiercinski, A. (2019). Hans-Georg Gadamer. In G. Stanghellini, M. R. Broome, A. V. Fernandez, P. Fusar-Poli, A. Raballo, & R. Rosfort (Eds.), *Oxford handbook of phenomenological psychopathology* (pp. 63–71). Oxford: Oxford University Press.

Ziv-Beiman, S., & Shahar, G. (2014). What is integrative psychotherapy? *Conversations: Israeli Journal of Psychotherapy, 28*(2), 156–163.

Concluding Remarks

Aner Govrin and Yael Peri Herzovich

Our book emerged from an extraordinary three-day gathering at Bar-Ilan University in September 2022, where 12 distinguished psychotherapists and scholars from different theoretical orientations came together to explore the possibility of meaningful dialogue across therapeutic divides. This workshop, titled "A Psychodynamic therapist and a CBT therapist meet on a plane... – Psychotherapy Integration as Hospitality," served as a living laboratory for examining how practitioners from different therapeutic traditions might engage productively with each other while maintaining their distinct professional identities.

Throughout these three days, we witnessed both the challenges and possibilities of cross-theoretical dialogue. We observed how discussions repeatedly circled back to fundamental questions of identity and legitimacy – psychoanalysts defending their approaches' scientific validity, cognitive-behavioral therapy (CBT) practitioners questioning the empirical basis of psychoanalytic concepts, each group struggling to maintain their professional identity while engaging with different perspectives. These interactions revealed that the barrier to integration lies not primarily in theoretical incompatibility or empirical disagreement but in the profound challenge of encountering professional "otherness" without feeling one's own professional identity threatened.

This realization led us to seek philosophical frameworks that might help us understand and potentially bridge these divides. We found that conventional arguments for integration – appeal to pragmatic effectiveness or theoretical pluralism – failed to address the deeper psychological and cultural barriers to meaningful dialogue between therapeutic schools. What was needed was a more sophisticated understanding of how therapeutic approaches might engage with each other while maintaining their distinct identities.

Drawing from our philosophical investigation, we developed three interrelated perspectives for understanding and facilitating therapeutic dialogue: hospitality (based on Derrida's work), dialectics (drawing on Hegel), and dialogue (inspired by Gadamer). Each of these perspectives illuminates different aspects of the challenge while suggesting practical paths forward.

Derrida's concept of hospitality proved particularly relevant to our workshop experiences. Just as hospitality involves welcoming strangers while maintaining

DOI: 10.4324/9781003608103-7

control over one's home, we observed how therapeutic approaches might host ideas from other orientations while maintaining their essential character. The tension Derrida describes between unconditional welcome and necessary limitations helped us understand how therapeutic schools might engage with other approaches while preserving their distinct identities.

Our exploration of Hegelian dialectics revealed how therapeutic approaches often develop through complex relationships with what they ostensibly reject. We witnessed this during the workshop as practitioners discovered how their own approaches had unconsciously incorporated elements they claimed to reject in others. This understanding helps explain why integration often occurs despite conscious resistance, and suggests ways to make this process more conscious and productive.

The concept of dialogue, as developed by Gadamer, helped us understand how the very differences that seem to block communication between therapeutic approaches might actually hold the key to deeper understanding. We saw this principle in action during workshop discussions where practitioners from different orientations found their understanding of their own approach enriched through engagement with different perspectives.

Throughout our investigation, we maintained focus on practical applications. Our workshop demonstrated that meaningful dialogue across theoretical boundaries is possible when approached with appropriate attitudes. We saw how practitioners from different orientations could engage productively when they felt their professional identities were respected and when clear boundaries were maintained.

The implications of our work extend beyond the specific case of psychoanalytic and cognitive-behavioral approaches. The frameworks we develop offer tools for thinking about integration across other therapeutic divides, relationships between clinical practice and research, and even the therapeutic relationship itself. Our experience suggests that acknowledging and working with identity threats, rather than ignoring them, may be key to productive integration between therapeutic approaches.

Our book does not argue for dissolving theoretical differences or suggest that all therapeutic approaches are equally valid. Instead, we propose frameworks for productive engagement across theoretical divides while maintaining rigorous standards of evaluation. We believe this represents a significant advance over both uncritical eclecticism and rigid theoretical purism.

What makes our contribution unique is its grounding in both philosophical sophistication and practical experience. The workshop provided a testing ground for our ideas about therapeutic dialogue, while our philosophical investigation helped us understand and articulate what we observed. The result is a framework that can help practitioners from different therapeutic orientations engage more productively with each other while maintaining their distinct professional identities.

On a more personal note, our experience organizing and participating in the three-day workshop profoundly influenced our understanding of therapeutic dialogue and professional growth. As we watched distinguished practitioners from different orientations struggle with and ultimately transcend their initial resistances, we witnessed something remarkable: moments of genuine openness and discovery that occurred precisely because of, rather than despite, theoretical differences.

What struck us most powerfully was how the most passionate defenders of their respective approaches – those most fascinated by their theoretical orientations – often had the most to gain from genuine engagement with other perspectives. We observed that deep commitment to one's theoretical approach, when combined with careful perpsectives for engaging with difference, could lead to particularly rich insights. It was often those most deeply versed in their own traditions who could most appreciate the subtle distinctions and contributions of other approaches.

Index

For Product Safety Concerns and Information please contact our EU
representative GPSR@taylorandfrancis.com
Taylor & Francis Verlag GmbH, Kaufingerstraße 24, 80331 München, Germany

www.ingramcontent.com/pod-product-compliance
Lightning Source LLC
Chambersburg PA
CBHW070350270326
41926CB00017B/4072